CANINE AND FELINE GERIATRICS

LIBRARY OF VETERINARY PRACTICE

EDITORS

J. B. SUTTON JP, MRCVS

S. T. SWIFT MA, VetMB, CertSAC

LIBRARY OF VETERINARY PRACTICE

CANINE AND FELINE GERIATRICS

MIKE DAVIES BVetMed, CertVR, CertSAO, FRCVS

**Blackwell
Science**

© 1996 by
Blackwell Science Ltd
Editorial Offices:
Osney Mead, Oxford OX2 0EL
25 John Street, London WC1N 2BL
23 Ainslie Place, Edinburgh EH3 6AJ
238 Main Street, Cambridge
  Massachusetts 02142, USA
54 University Street, Carlton
  Victoria 3053, Australia

Other Editorial Offices:
Arnette Blackwell SA
  224, Boulevard Saint Germain
  75007 Paris, France

Blackwell Wissenschafts-Verlag GmbH
  Kurfürstendamm 57
  10707 Berlin, Germany

  Zehetnergasse 6
  A-1140 Wien
  Austria

First published 1996

Set in 10.5/13pt Souvenir
by DP Photosetting, Aylesbury, Bucks
Printed and bound in Great Britain

The Blackwell Science logo is a trade mark of
Blackwell Science Ltd, registered at the United
Kingdom Trade Marks Registry

DISTRIBUTORS

Marston Book Services Ltd
PO Box 269
Abingdon
Oxon OX14 4YN
(*Orders:* Tel: 01235 465500
        Fax: 01235 465555)

USA
Blackwell Science, Inc.
238 Main Street
Cambridge, MA 02142
(*Orders:* Tel: 800 215-1000
        617 876-7000
        Fax: 617 492-5263)

Canada
Copp Clark, Ltd
2775 Matheson Blvd East
Mississauga, Ontario
Canada, L4W 4P7
(*Orders:* Tel: 800 263-4374
        905 238-6074)

Australia
Blackwell Science Pty Ltd
54 University Street
Carlton, Victoria 3053
(*Orders:* Tel: 03 9347 0300
        Fax: 03 9349 3016)

A catalogue record for this title
is available from the British Library

ISBN 0–632–03479–3

Library of Congress
Cataloging-in-Publication Data
Davies, Mike.
    Canine and feline geriatrics/Mike Davies.
      p.   cm. – (Library of veterinary
practice)
    Includes bibliographical references and
index.
      ISBN 0–632–03479–3 (pbk.)
      1. Dogs—Aging.   2. Dogs—Diseases.
    3. Cats—Aging.   4. Cats—Diseases.
    5. Veterinary geriatrics.   I. Title.
    II. Series.
    SF991.D37   1996
    636.7′089897—dc20   96–20438
                                        CIP

CONTENTS

PREFACE

At the time of writing this book the study of geriatrics as a veterinary discipline is very much in its infancy. My interest in the subject is obviously becoming more acute as I work through my own midlife crises and see old age looming on the not-too-distant horizon, but the main stimulus for me to write this book came from Dr J. Mosier (USA), a pioneer of the study of geriatrics in veterinary medicine, and Dr Mary Harrington, a human geriatrician in London – both of whom took part in a Symposium on Geriatric Veterinary Medicine which I organised in London in 1988.

In researching for this book I was disappointed at the relative lack of published work on many aspects of geriatrics in veterinary medicine. However I am pleased to say that there is now a considerable amount of work going on – particularly in the areas of progressive renal disease and cognitive disorders. There are inherent dangers in extrapolating too much from experimental studies and from studies conducted in different species, nevertheless there are many useful comparative correlations to be drawn from veterinary species to humans and vice versa.

Much work needs to be done to obtain base information about geriatric veterinary patients and in the meantime it would be helpful to the development of veterinary geriatric medicine if the non-sensitive research data from studies in cats and dogs currently held by many pharmaceutical companies and other institutions could be made available.

I have tried to draw together relevant information from the published (and unpublished) works of many researchers in various fields and I wish to thank them for documenting their subjects so well. I have tried to make sense out of the information available and to address some of the main issues in geriatric medicine to assist clinicians in first opinion practice. I have avoided in-depth coverage of some topics such as arthritis which perhaps should be in a book on geriatrics, but these are well documented in other publications.

At times I have been deliberately controversial and I look forward to receiving correspondence from colleagues with alternative views!

I have absolutely no doubt that this book will need to be totally revised within the next few years but in the meantime I hope that it will stimulate some of my colleagues to look further at this interesting group of patients which present such a clinical challenge, and I hope that it may lead to an improvement in the future care and management of geriatric veterinary patients.

Mike Davies BVetMed CertVR CertSAO FRCVS
Dorset, March 1996

ACKNOWLEDGEMENT

Plate 7 was reproduced courtesy of B.D. Murdoch.

Chapter 1

AN INTRODUCTION TO GERIATRIC VETERINARY MEDICINE

1.1 INTRODUCTION

Great advances have been made in human geriatric medicine over the past 20 years. Old people are now regarded as a separate clinical group from the young adult population, and the development of specialisation in 'geriatrics' has increased our knowledge of many of the diseases of the elderly and so improved their treatment and management.

Old people are often reluctant to seek medical attention early in the course of a disease, believing that their illness is simply due to 'old age' and that nothing can be done for them. In veterinary practice we face a similar problem because pet owners often do not present an animal when it develops mild signs of disease such as increased thirst or increased frequency of urination in the belief that such signs are an inevitable result of advancing age.

Farm animals and some groups of working dogs are not allowed to survive to old age and for these animals there is little available information about the effects of ageing. The oldest recorded age for a horse is 62 years and for a cow 78 years (Matthews 1994). The oldest recorded cat was 34 years, and the oldest dog 29 years, but most dogs live for 8–15 years with large and giant breeds having a shorter life expectancy than small breeds (Matthews 1994). Pet owners (including breeders) sometimes prefer to terminate their animals' lives early rather than allow them to attain their full life expectancy and have to support them through old age.

Some owners delay presenting an old animal for treatment because of a genuine fear that the veterinarian might detect a serious illness and advise euthanasia. In fact, most diseases of the aged can be treated and, even if not curable, something can usually be done to improve the quality of life for the animal. If an animal does have a terminal condition, delaying a visit to the veterinary surgeon is not going to help matters, and in the meantime the individual could be subject to unnecessary suffering.

One of the most significant advances in human geriatric medicine has been the introduction of routine screening tests. These have brought to the fore a whole spectrum of diseases originally thought to be rare, but now known to be common. Routine screening improves the identification of risk factors and the early detection of disease allowing early intervention and, as a result, patients are living longer, and the mean life-expectancy of the population as a whole is increasing.

Undoubtedly similar advances will be made in veterinary geriatrics, particularly in the area of preventative medicine and the identification and avoidance of risk factors.

1.2 THE DEMOGRAPHICS OF GERIATRIC CATS AND DOGS

In human medicine a large amount of actuarial information has been collected over many years by the insurance companies, and their increasing need to identify risk factors for disease is greatly improving the application of early screening and interpretation of results. The overall effect of these measures is to increase mean longevity by helping people to recognise and avoid risk factors such as obesity, high cholesterol intake, smoking, drugs and alcohol abuse.

In 1988 approximately 5% of the human population living in western civilisation were estimated to be over retirement age. In the UK 17% of people were over retirement age and this is anticipated to rise to above 20% by the year 2000 (Harrington 1988). In the USA it was estimated that 17% of dogs and cats were 'geriatric' (i.e. dogs over 10 years, cats over 12 years of age) (Mosier 1988).

A 'Market Facts Study' conducted in the USA in 1984 produced the following figures for animals presenting to veterinary surgeries:

Dogs

1 year old or less	16%
2-5 years	41%
6 years or more	43%

Cats

1 year old or less	25%
2–5 years	44%
6 years or more	31%

In the UK a survey of 6417 cats and 20 786 dogs presented to the Small Animal Practice Teaching Unit (SAPTU) at Edinburgh University (1991) revealed the following figures for animals presented to them for first and second opinion services:

Dogs

Less than 1 year of age	19.4%
1–6 years	45.7%
7 years or more	34.9%

Cats

Less than 1 year of age	32.1%
1–6 years	40%
7 years or more	27.9%

Hence a significant number of animals presented to a veterinary surgery are in the 'old age' category.

The age distributions of dogs and cats from the SAPTU survey are shown in Figs 1.1 and 1.2.

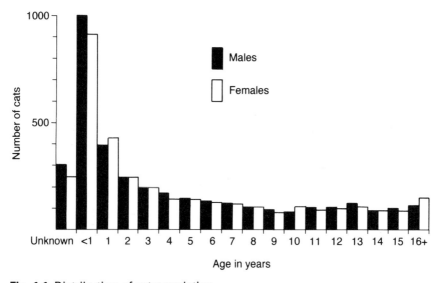

Fig. 1.1 Distribution of cat population

1.3 DEFINING THE TERM 'GERIATRIC'

Dictionaries define 'geriatric' as 'pertaining to old people' and the World Health Organization (1963) has defined 'middle-age' as being 45–59 years, 'elderly' as being 60–74 years and the 'aged' as over 75 years of

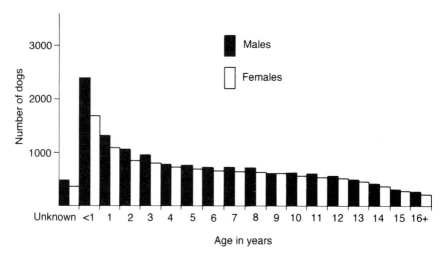

Fig. 1.2 Distribution of dog population

age. In human terms the elderly should be regarded by society as a useful resource because of their knowledge, skills and experience but the aged most often need assistance. Unfortunately there is no similar classification for our domesticated species and there is no specific definition of a geriatric animal, though we all recognise external signs of increasing age such as greying of the muzzle, stiffness in movement, changes in posture, reduced responsiveness to outside stimuli, and so on.

There are many problems about defining life-stages based on chronological age in cats and dogs because breeds have differing rates of ageing, lead different life-styles and have different life expectancies. I would therefore like to propose a simplified classification scheme (Table 1.1) based upon functionality rather than chronological age which can be applied at any time to any individual.

There are many theories about the ageing process including the concept that all living creatures are genetically programmed to age – a 'biological clock' theory. Most higher living organisms have a relatively brief life consisting of the following basic life stages: conception, growth, reproduction and death. Only a few species (including humans and domesticated pets) pass through a post-reproductive senescent stage known as 'old age'. In the wild, most animals have predators that prevent the frail and infirm from surviving.

The ageing process is complex and we have yet to discover its secret. The person who does – and can find a way to delay it – stands to make a fortune!

In humans, the mean life-expectancy can be predicted based upon sex,

Table 1.1 Proposed description for age stages of cats and dogs.

Age stage	Description
1 (Fetal)	Conception to birth – from fertilisation through embryological development to birth
2 (Growth)	Growth – from birth until skeletal growth is completed
3 (Adulthood)	Young adulthood – active reproductive phase. Until age-related changes affect appearance and/or organ function
6 (Ageing)	Advanced adulthood – obvious external signs of ageing and/or evidence of age-related changes affecting the function of at least one major organ system
7 (Senile)	Age-related loss of central nervous system function leading to cognitive impairment and/or loss of control over at least one major organ system

race, socio-economic and other factors. For example, in Western society women live longer than men and smokers have a reduced life expectancy. Factors affecting the life expectancy of cats and dogs have not been fully determined and within breed and across-breed comparisons have not been made though it is generally accepted that large and giant breeds of dog have a shorter life expectancy than small breeds.

1.4 AGEING CHANGES

We can make several observations about ageing changes:

(1) they are progressive
(2) they are irreversible
(3) multiple organ systems are involved
(4) physiological mechanisms ultimately become impaired
(5) variable expression is shown between individuals.

Ageing changes that may occur in tissues include:

- atrophy
- fatty infiltration
- fibrosis
- delayed ability to repair
- reduced number of active cells
- reduced rate of activity
- reduced organ function.

The pigment lipofuscin is deposited in body tissues in increasing amounts with increasing age, indeed it has been called 'the pigment of ageing'. In the dog lipofuscin is deposited at five times the rate that it is in humans.

Ageing changes proceed at varying rates in different organ systems of the body, and may be present in varying degrees of severity between individuals of the same age. Typically, older animals lose sensitivity of their major senses, e.g. vision, hearing, taste and smell, and all organ systems may be affected to some degree by age-related changes.

Geriatric screening is helpful in determining whether or not organ function is impaired, particularly before elective procedures such as minor surgery. Some organ systems are more likely to be affected than others, for example with increasing age teeth are likely to demonstrate:

- dental calculus accumulation
- gingival hyperplasia
- periodontitis
- gum atrophy and retraction
- enamel wear
- ulcerative lesions
- tooth loss.

By the time they are 7–8 years of age 95% of dogs are said to be affected by periodontal disease (Harvey 1988).

The occurrence of obesity increases with age probably due to:

(1) reduced lean body mass (hence reduced basal energy requirement (BER))
(2) reduced exercise
(3) overnutrition.

Obesity can have serious effects on other body systems, e.g. cardiovascular and skeletal systems, and may have a role in the cause of some diseases, e.g. diabetes mellitus.

Some age-related changes that may be seen in various organ systems are listed below (after Mosier and others):

Gastrointestinal tract

- reduced salivary secretion
- impaired oesophageal function (neuronal)
- reduced HCl secretion
- slower rate of renewal of epithelium
- reduced villous size
- impaired nutrient absorption.

Liver

- decreased number of hepatocytes
- increased binucleated hepatocytes
- fatty infiltration
- increased fibrous tissue
- decreased hepatic function
- decreased bile formation.

Kidney

- reduced renal size
- reduced number of nephrons
- reduced glomerular filtration rate (GFR)
- reduced renal plasma flow
- reduced tubular excretion
- reduced tubular reabsorption.

Eye

- iris atrophy
- nuclear sclerosis
- cataracts
- loss of rods and cones
- cystoid retinal degeneration
- asteroid hyalosis
- eyelid papillomas
- cysts of the gland of Moll
- increased tear viscosity
- decreased lysozyme activity, increased susceptibility to infection
- corneal pigment changes due chronic irritation.

Skin

- hair becomes sparse, dull and lustreless
- patchy alopecia
- white hairs (loss of pigment)
- calluses over pressure points
- skin thickens, reduced pliability
- hyperkeratosis; later, epidermis atrophies
- calcium/pseudoelastin replace elastic fibres
- hyperplasia of apocrine and sebaceous glands.

Endocrine system

- fatty infiltration, cyst formation and fibrosis
- reduced hormone production, e.g. thyroid and sex hormones
- reduced response to T3 and T4
- reduced T4 binding capacity of serum proteins
- chronic thyroiditis (15–20% aged beagles)
- reduced response to adrenocorticotrophic hormone (ACTH)
- mammary nodules/tumours in 80% intact bitches at 11 years age.

Skeletal system

- loss of muscle mass
- reduced number and size of muscle cells
- fibrosis, atrophy and reduced response to adenosine triphosphate (ATP)
- impaired resynthesis of ATP
- impaired ability to use amino acids as an energy source
- reduced oxygen transport
- reduced neuromuscular function
- long bone cortices thin, change in density and become brittle
- reduced number and activity of osteoblasts
- reduced amount of cartilage which splits and fragments
- reduced mucopolysaccharide production
- reduced chondroitin sulphate production
- spondylosis and costochondral calcification
- degenerative joint disease
- synovial fluid thickens with increased globulin content
- increased rheumatoid and antinuclear factors.

Central nervous system

- neurotransmitter changes;
- acetylcholinesterase levels increase, choline acetyltransferase decreases;
- monoamine oxidase levels increase, causing decreased neurotransmitter levels;
- reduced serotonin increases sleep, and causes neuromuscular disorders and depression;
- stimulation of interneurones in the brain is longer lasting, leading to short-term memory loss, impaired learning and delayed response time;

- hypoxia due to reduced respiratory function and cardiovascular changes, e.g. arteriocapillary fibrosis;
- senile behaviour changes, e.g. loss of house training.

Peripheral nervous system

- loss of reflexes;
- cell loss and lipofuscin accumulation in ganglia of sympathetic and parasympathetic systems cause impaired gut motility (constipation);
- reduced reaction to stimuli and partial loss of senses (taste, vision, hearing and smell).

Respiratory system

- obstructive lung disease
- reduced ciliary activity
- decreased secretions with increased viscosity
- bronchial constriction due to decreased adenosine monophosphate (cAMP)
- pulmonary fibrosis
- decreased alveolar diffusing capacity
- depressed cough reflex
- chronic bronchitis
- hypoxaemia.

Immune system

- involution of lymph nodes, Peyer's patches and tonsils
- reduced size of cortices in lymph nodes
- reduced immunocompetence despite normal numbers of immunocytes.

Haematology

- bone marrow becomes pale and fatty
- splenomegaly with hyperplasia, haemosiderosis and haematomas
- decreased red blood cell count and haemoglobin carrying capacity
- relative anaemia (common)
- replenishment of red cells may take longer (2 ×).

These types of age-related changes may impair normal physiological activities, reduce the ability of the animal to respond to stresses, infections or other attacks on the body, and delay healing processes. Nevertheless advanced age is not regarded as being a disease state.

Because of reduced hepatic function, renal function and suboptimal metabolic processes older animals may have an impaired ability to metabolise and excrete drugs. Hence medications may need to be given at different dose rates from the normal adult dose. There may also be additional risks associated with general anaesthesia or elective surgery.

1.5   GERIATRIC DISEASES

Geriatric disease can be classified (Harrington 1988) as:

(1) diseases proper to old age
(2) diseases that persist into old age
(3) diseases with a changing incidence in old age.

In many cases of frank clinical disease in older animals there will be concurrent problems affecting other body systems (Mosier 1988). No two clinical cases in geriatric animals are exactly the same (Mosier 1988).

Many of the diseases that appear in old age are chronic and insidious, often being present for many months or even years before the owner notices signs. Subclinical disease may present serious difficulties in managing a case.

Advancing age is, in itself, a risk factor for the development of certain diseases, e.g. neoplasia, acute renal failure, endocardiosis.

The objectives of management of a geriatric animal are:

(1) prevent or delay the onset of disease
(2) identify and ameliorate existing problems as early as possible
(3) maintain body weight and condition
(4) maintain quality of life.

Prolongation of life is not, in itself, a valid clinical objective if the animal will suffer as a result of intervention and its quality of life is poor.

REFERENCES AND FURTHER READING

Anon. (1984) *Market Facts Study.* Hill's Pet Products Inc.
Anon. (1989) Geriatrics and Gerontology. *Veterinary Clinics of North America: Small Animal Practice,* **19**(1).
Hamlin, R.L. (1987) Managing cardiologic disorders in geriatric dogs. In: *Geriatric Medicine: Contemporary Clinical and Practice Management Approaches.* pp. 14–18. Veterinary Medicine Publishing Company, Topeka, Kansas.
Harrington, M. (1988) The progress of geriatric medicine in the UK: a starting point for interdisciplinary dialogue. *Proceedings of Symposium on Clinical*

Conditions in the Older Cat and Dog, The Royal Garden Hotel, London, 15 June 1988. p. 4. Published by Hill's Pet Products, London.

Harvey, C.E. (1988) Oral diseases of ageing animals. *Proceedings of Symposium on Clinical Conditions in the Older Cat and Dog*, The Royal Garden Hotel, London, 15 June 1988. pp. 58–62. Published by Hill's Pet Products, London.

Lewis, L.D., Morris, M.L. & Hand, M.S. (1987) *Small Animal Clinical Nutrition III*. Mark Morris Associates, Topeka, Kansas.

Matthews, P. (ed.) (1994) *The New Guinness Book of Records 1995*. Guinness Publishing Ltd., Enfield.

Mosier, J.E. (1987) How aging affects body systems in the dog. In: *Geriatric Medicine: Contemporary Clinical and Practice Management Approaches*. pp. 2–5. Veterinary Medicine Publishing Company, Topeka, Kansas.

Mosier, J.E. (1988) *Proceedings of Symposium on Clinical Conditions in the Older Cat and Dog*, The Royal Garden Hotel, London, 15 June 1988. Published by Hill's Pet Products, London.

Pathy, M.S.J. (ed.) (1991) *Principles and Practice of Geriatric Medicine*, 2nd edn. John Wiley, Chichester.

Special Symposium on Canine Geriatric Medicine. Published in *Veterinary Medicine*, May 1990.

Valtonen, M.H. (1972) Cardiovascular disease and nephritis in dogs. *Journal of Small Animal Practice*, **13**, 687–97.

Whitney, J.C. (1974) Observations on the effect of age on the severity of heart valve lesions in the dog. *Journal of Small Animal Practice*, **15**, 511–22.

World Health Organization (1963) *Report of a Seminar on the Health Protection of the Elderly and Aged and the Prevention of Premature Ageing*. WHO Regional Office in Europe, Copenhagen.

Chapter 2
THE CARDIOVASCULAR SYSTEM

KEY POINTS

(1) Cardiovascular disease is very common in old dogs.
(2) Heart disease is often subclinical and the onset of heart failure insidious.
(3) The incidence and severity of chronic valvular lesions increase with advancing age in dogs.
(4) Concurrent disease in other organ systems is common.
(5) Except for Stage IV emergency cases, a full physical examination is necessary to confirm the presence of concomitant disease before specific therapy is started.
(6) Minimise the exposure of geriatric animals to cardiovascular risk factors such as obesity and high dietary salt intake.

2.1 REDUCED CARDIOVASCULAR FUNCTION

The cardiovascular system is the most important organ system in the body because maintenance of blood flow to and from cells is essential for the normal function and survival of all body tissues. When cardiovascular function is impaired it has deleterious effects on many organ systems, including the cardiovascular system itself.

Reduced tissue perfusion

Reduced tissue perfusion may result in:

(1) hypoxia
(2) poor cell nutrition
(3) reduced supply of immune mediators
(4) failure to remove metabolic waste products and toxins
(5) failure to transport physiologically active substances.

Compensatory mechanisms

In the presence of reduced cardiac function compensatory mechanisms come into operation which attempt to maintain blood flow to vital organs such as the brain and heart, and in the process blood may be diverted away from other tissues such as the abdominal viscera. These haemodynamic changes are helpful in hypovolaemia or shock and may have no serious consequences in the short-term for healthy individuals, but they can be deleterious when maintained over a long period of time, particularly in elderly animals in which tissues may be more susceptible to the adverse effects of reduced or increased perfusion.

Many ageing dogs have cardiovascular lesions but they are in a stable, compensated state with perhaps an audible murmur but no signs of heart failure. Veterinary cardiologists traditionally do not recommend therapeutic intervention until the animal is decompensated and clinical signs of failure are present, but it is important to realise that the compensatory mechanisms themselves may have adverse effects on the body. Prolonged sympathetic stimulation, for example, may induce insulin resistance and reduce glucose tolerance, with important metabolic consequences for the individual.

Cardiac workload

One objective in the management of geriatric animals with clinical or sub-clinical heart disease should be to reduce unnecessary workload on the heart. The sum of the forces acting upon the myocardium to stretch the muscle fibres at the end of diastole is called the preload, and the sum of the forces opposing myocardial contraction during systole is called the after-load.

Restriction of dietary salt intake is one simple mechanism by which preload can be decreased, and avoidance or reduction of obesity can also significantly reduce cardiac workload. In the presence of clinical disease therapeutic agents such as diuretics can be used to reduce preload and vasodilators to modify preload and afterload.

Secondary heart disease

Control of cardiac activity depends upon the normal function and co-ordination of several organ systems including the peripheral nervous system (sympathetic and parasympathetic), endocrine function (e.g. adrenal and thyroid), the cardiovascular system itself and the metabolic state of the animal (e.g. electrolyte balance, acid–base balance).

Various chemical agents, toxins, nutritional abnormalities (deficiencies, excesses or imbalances), systemic diseases or metabolic diseases parti-cularly those of the liver, kidneys, lungs or endocrine system may interfere with cardiovascular function causing secondary heart disease.

Concomitant disease

In geriatric patients presenting with cardiac disease it is important to consider the likelihood of concomitant disorders in other organ systems:

(1) as a primary cause of the heart disease, e.g. hyperthyroidism;
(2) secondary to the heart disease, e.g. reduced renal function;
(3) reducing the efficacy of therapeutic agents, e.g. reduced efficacy of diuretics in the presence of hypoproteinaemia associated with reduced liver function;
(4) enhancing the toxicity of therapeutic agents, e.g. digoxin toxicity in the presence of renal failure or hypokalaemia.

2.2   AGE-RELATED TISSUE CHANGES

Structural changes

Structural changes found with increasing age which may or may not be associated with clinical signs of disease include:

Heart

- valvular thickening (fibrosis)
- myocardial fibrosis
- myocardial necrosis
- microscopic coronary arteriosclerosis
- microscopic intramural myocardial infarction (MIMIs)
- myocardial hypertrophy*
- fatty infiltration
- chamber dilatation*
- lipofuscin accumulation in myocyte cytoplasm

- Myocardial amyloid deposition.
  * Compensatory changes

Lipofuscin accumulation in myocyte cytoplasm increases with age in the dog, and starts at about 7 years of age. It is not known whether it has any adverse effect on myocyte function.

Cardiac amyloidosis is a frequent finding at post-mortem examination in geriatric humans (50% of people over 65 years, and 84% of people over 90 years), but in one study of dogs only 0.6% (all over 10 years of age) had this change at routine autopsy.

In one report valvular endocardiosis lesions increased in incidence and severity with increasing age, and were present in all dogs over 13 years of age (Whitney 1974).

Blood vessels

- arteriosclerosis
- fibrous thickening of the intima or media of the aorta
- hyaline or amyloid thickening of the media of blood vessels
- calcification of the aortic intima
- calcification of the media in peripheral vessels
- muscular hypertrophy of small and medium-sized arterioles
- arteriocapillary fibrosis
- increased capillary fragility
- increased capillary permeability
- atherosclerosis – rare compared with man.

Arteriosclerosis of intramural coronary arteries has been reported to occur in 77.6% of geriatric dogs over 12 years of age (Valtonen 1972), 60% of dogs over 14 years of age (Detweiler *et al.* 1968) and 50% of dogs aged 13 years or older (Jonsson 1972). A direct association was found between the presence of arteriosclerosis and microscopic intramural myocardial infarcts (MIMIs).

These structural changes cause a loss of elasticity of vascular walls and/ or luminal narrowing, and contribute to increased peripheral resistance which, combined with reduced sensitivity to the vasodilator effect of β-adrenergic stimulation (see below), probably contributes to the increased aortic impedance and left ventricular afterload seen in geriatric patients.

Vessels supplying various organs throughout the body may be affected, notably the kidney and brain, resulting in impaired vascular supply, and ultimately impaired organ function.

Atherosclerosis leading to myocardial infarction while common in humans is rare in dogs and cats. Obesity and thyroid atrophy or frank hypothyroidism are associated with the development of atherosclerosis in geriatric dogs. Experimentally, atherosclerosis can only be caused in hypothyroid dogs on high fat diets. Miniature schnauzers with hyperlipidaemia may be predisposed to develop atherosclerosis.

Metabolic changes

Metabolic changes reported to occur in the cardiovascular system with increasing age include changes in myocardial enzymes:

(1) monoamine oxidase and malic deshydrogenase activity increase
(2) dopamine β-oxidase, dopa decarboxylase, lactic dehydrogenase, cytochrome oxidase and glucose-6-phosphate dehydrogenase activity decrease.

Cardiac performance with increasing age

Changes in cardiac performance with increasing age have been reported in dogs. Older (8–12 years old) beagles were found to have a reduced maximum heart rate in response to isoproterenol administration than younger (1–4 years old) beagles (Yin *et al.* 1979). Also, increased impedance to left ventricular ejection has been demonstrated at exercise in 10–14-year-old beagles compared with younger individuals (Yin *et al.* 1981) demonstrating that ventricular afterload increases in older dogs.

These changes are thought to be caused by reduced cardiovascular response to β-adrenergic stimulation due to uncoupling of an intracellular pathway possibly related to cyclic AMP or protein kinase phosphorylation. Receptor sensitivity is reduced in the presence of catecholamines, and increased catecholamine concentrations have been reported in old people, who develop similar reductions in function. Chronically increased catecholamine concentrations also occur as one of the physiological mechanisms in cardiac compensation, such as in response to reduced cardiac output in endocardiosis.

Reduced response to β-adrenergic stimulation in the peripheral vasculature decreases vasodilation which was demonstrated in the study of beagles at exercise (Yin *et al.* 1981) as the lower impedance in the young dogs was eliminated by administration of beta-blocker.

Myocyte contraction and relaxation times are prolonged with increasing age, a phenomenon thought to be due to reduced uptake of calcium ions by the sarcoplasmic reticulum, resulting in increased contact time between the calcium and actin and myosin filaments. In rats reduced concentrations of the enzyme calcium adenosinetriphosphatase have been reported, which might explain such an effect.

There is one report that cardiac output in dogs decreases by 30% from the middle to last one-third of a dog's lifespan (Mosier 1987). However, there are conflicting reports from human studies about this effect of ageing and currently it is thought that cardiac output is probably maintained at rest, but left ventricular ejection fraction is reduced in elderly human patients during exercise. In other words the cardiovascular system of geriatric patients has difficulty in adapting to increased workloads, reinforcing the need to minimise exposure to excessive workload.

2.3 DIAGNOSTIC AIDS

Accurate diagnosis depends on careful consideration of the history and physical examination. In geriatric patients the minimum database should also include some basic clinical tests including packed cell volume, total protein, urinalysis, survey chest radiography, electrocardiogram (ECG) and sometimes echocardiography.

Radiography

Left atrial enlargement can be seen on a dorsoventral view as a bulge at the 2–3 o'clock position, and on the lateral view there is separation of the mainstem bronchi with the left bronchus being forced dorsally.

Left ventricular enlargement is recognised on a lateral view by straightening of the caudal border of the heart, sometimes becoming convex, and loss of the caudal cardiac 'waist'. The trachea is elevated dorsally and the presence of pulmonary venous congestion is recognised by enlargement of pulmonary veins, and the presence of pulmonary oedema (interstitial and/or alveolar), particularly in the perihilar region of the lung field.

Right atrial enlargement is recognised on the lateral view by cranial bulging of the cardiac silhouette, and on the dorsoventral view by bulging at the 10 o'clock position. The trachea is elevated over the cranial part of the heart on the lateral view.

On a lateral view right ventricular enlargement causes increased sternal contact and increased convexity of the cranial border of the cardiac silhouette. The apex of the heart is sometimes lifted off the sternum. The trachea is elevated over the cranial heart.

Right-sided heart failure results in passive venous congestion of abdominal structures and radiographic evidence of hepatomegaly, splenomegaly and ascites are often present as well as enlargement of the caudal vena cava. If there is underperfusion of the lung, pulmonary arteries and veins may appear thin and the lung parenchyma radiolucent.

A large rounded cardiac silhouette is indicative of pericardial effusion (though in younger animals peritoneopericardial diaphragmatic hernias or per cardial cysts may give a similar radiographic appearance). Positive contrast studies using an image intensifier may be useful to demonstrate valvular regurgitation during systole.

Echocardiography

M-mode echocardiography is a superior imaging method to radiography because abnormal morphology of the valves can be visualised, and chamber dimensions and contractility can be measured.

Doppler, in particular colour flow Doppler, is extremely useful in detecting blood flow abnormalities associated with valvular regurgitation.

Electrocardiography

An ECG is essential if an arrhythmia is detected on auscultation but may not be particularly helpful in some cases, e.g. chronic valvular endo-cardiosis.

Left atrial enlargement may cause a prolonged P wave (greater than 0.04 s in both the dog and cat) called P mitrale. Prolonged P waves may be biphasic.

Right atrial enlargement (seen with tricuspid insufficiency) may cause an increased P wave voltage (greater than 0.4 mV in the dog, greater than 0.2 mV in the cat) called P pulmonale. Both P pulmonale and P mitrale may be present at the same time.

Left ventricular enlargement may result in tall R waves, and prolonged QRS complexes. Slurring of the ST segment may be seen.

Right ventricular enlargement may result in right axis deviation and deep S waves (greater than 0.35 mV in lead II), and positive T waves in lead V 10.

Notching of the QRS complex (R wave) is often seen in geriatric dogs and is thought to be caused by the presence of MIMIs.

Laboratory screening

In the author's opinion routine laboratory screening of geriatric dogs with heart disease is mandatory, particularly before the administration of drugs which might be hepatotoxic or nephrotoxic such as the cardiac glycosides.

Chronic diuretic use may induce hypokalaemia, indeed hypokalaemia is probably common but rarely detected because it is not routinely screened for. Elevated liver enzymes are likely to be detected if hepatic congestion is present, and prerenal azotaemia is common in the presence of reduced cardiac output.

2.4   GERIATRIC CARDIOVASCULAR DISEASE

Some cats and dogs with congenital heart disorders may survive into old age, as will many animals that develop clinical signs of heart disease in middle-age. Successful management of these cases through old age requires an understanding of the physical, metabolic and systemic changes that the individuals are undergoing due to normal ageing changes and concurrent organ disease. Destabilisation may occur, and readjustment of drug doses may be needed in some individuals, particularly those that develop signs of decompensation or drug toxicity.

Clinical conditions that would normally be expected to occur earlier in life may appear for the first time in old age, but in this section we shall only consider those cardiovascular diseases which are normally expected to occur in geriatric patients.

1.   Acquired chronic valvular disease (endocardiosis)

Incidence

Acquired atrioventricular valvular endocardiosis is the most common canine heart condition accounting for over 70% of cases, with a reported overall incidence of 17–40%. The disease is most prevalent in small to medium size dogs in the last third of their life, males are more often affected than females (1.5 : 1) and it increases both in frequency and severity with increasing age.

One study reported severe disease to be present in 58% of dogs over 9 years of age, and endocardiosis lesions were present in all dogs over 13 years of age (Whitney 1974). The author concluded that the frequency of occurrence and the severity of the valvular lesions increased with increasing age (Tables 2.1 and 2.2).

Endocardiosis is rarely reported in cats.

Table 2.1 Frequency of AV lesions in 200 canine hearts (Whitney 1974).

	0–4 years age	5–8 years age	9–12 years age	13–16 years age
Left AV valve (% frequency of lesions)	37%	80%	93%	100%

Table 2.2 Percentage frequency of left AV valve lesions according to severity grade of endocardiosis (Whitney 1974).

Type	0–4 years age	5–8 years age	9–12 years age	13–16 years age
I	15	28	12	7
II	13	38	29	7
III	9	20	33	34
IV	0	3	20	54

Aetiopathogenesis

The cause of the valvular lesions seen in endocardiosis is unknown, but natural ageing processes have been suggested by some authors, either:

(1) associated with ageing changes in the collagen fibres of the valves, or
(2) valve injury progressing to a degenerative lesion.

It is commonly believed that chronic valvular disease begins in the first third of life, progresses to cause valvular incompetence in the second third of life, and may be associated with congestive heart failure in the last third of life, though most dogs are likely to develop cardiac compensation and not progress to exhibit clinical signs of failure.

Gross lesions

Greyish-white nodules or plaques on the valves, with weakening and thickening of the chordae tendinae. Jet lesions on the atrium.

Lesions most often involve the left atrioventricular valve (mitral) and less commonly the right atrioventricular (tricuspid) valve (see Plate 1). The aortic and pulmonary valves are rarely affected.

Histopathology

Various changes have been described including:

(1) myxomatous changes
(2) deposition of hyaline (fibrinoid) material

(3) fibrous and elastic proliferation
(4) mucoid degeneration.

There is proliferation of the spongiosa layer of the valve with increased amounts of matrix containing glycosaminoglycans (GAGs).

Pathophysiology

The valvular lesions result in:

 (1) inadequate closure of the valves during systole with regurgitation of blood into the atrium
 (2) volume overload of atrium and ventricule
 (3) compensatory atrial and ventricular dilatation
 (4) myocardial hypertrophy
 (5) myocardial failure (eventually)
 (6) pulmonary oedema (due to pulmonary vein compression)
 (7) left mainstem bronchus compression (causes a cough)
 (8) bronchoconstriction (if pulmonary oedema present)
 (9) dysrhythmias (due to stretching of chamber wall)
(10) rupture of the atrium with haemopericardium (rare)
(11) rupture of the chordae tendinae.

Endocardiosis results in 'backward' failure or left-sided heart failure initially.

History

Exercise intolerance and coughing are the most frequent owner complaints. Often there is a history of weight loss (even if the dog is still overweight).

Clinical findings

(1) systolic murmur present on auscultation, and localisable to the site of the mitral and/or tricuspid valve
(2) a precordial thrill may be palpable
(3) sinus tachycardia sometimes with dysrhythmias
(4) pulse deficit (sometimes).

Treatment

Preload reducers, e.g. salt restriction, diuretics and vasodilators. Cardiac inotropes, e.g. cardiac glycosides.

2.   Bacterial endocarditis

Incidence

Most commonly affects older, male, large breed dogs, and German shepherd dogs may be predisposed to develop the condition. It is rare in the cat.

Gross pathology

Large cauliflower-like vegetative masses develop attached to the endothelium of the valve leaflets. The mitral valve is most commonly affected, followed by the aortic valve. The tricuspid valve is only occasionally involved.

When bacterial endocarditis does occur in the cat is usually affects the mitral valve.

Histopathology

The lesions consist of bacteria, with inflammatory cells (mononuclear cells and neutrophils) and platelets in an amorphous mass of fibrin and necrotic tissues.

Aetiopathogenesis

Usually secondary to a bacteraemia. Bacteria most frequently cultured from the lesions are coagulase positive staphylococci (particularly *Staphylococcus aureus*), *Escherichia coli* and β-haemolytic streptococci. Periodontal infection is very common in older dogs and cats, and may act as a primary site for the development of a bacteraemia.

Emboli from the heart valves may travel to any organ, e.g. the kidney, spleen and myocardium, causing abscesses or infarction.

Pathophysiology

The lesions cause valvular regurgitation or incompetence, leading to left-sided heart failure.

Clinical findings

The most common clinical findings in decreasing order of occurrence are:

(1) fever
(2) tachycardia
(3) vomiting
(4) lameness
(5) cardiac murmur
(6) ventricular arrhythmia
(7) renal failure
(8) heart failure
(9) sudden death
(10) myopathy.

Laboratory findings

(1) positive blood culture – not always detected
(2) leukocytosis with left shift
(3) monocytosis
(4) low serum albumin
(5) increased serum alkaline phosphatase (occasional finding)
(6) hypoglycaemia (occasional finding)
(7) normocytic normochromic anaemia
(8) increased erythrocyte sedimentation rate.

Diagnosis

Is based on history and clinical signs, laboratory findings, the presence of a murmur and positive blood culture. Echocardiographic examination is also very helpful.

Treatment

Prolonged high dose bactericidal antibiotics (ideally based on culture and sensitivity results) which penetrate fibrin. Several antibiotics are usually given alternatively over a 6–8-week period.

S. aureus are usually:

Sensitive to	Resistant to
Cephalosporins	Penicillin
Aminoglycosides	Ampicillin
Erythromycin	Trimethoprim
Chloramphenicol	

E. coli are usually:

Sensitive to	Resistant to
Gentamicin	Ampicillin
Cephalosporins	Chloramphenicol

β-Haemolytic streptococci are usually:

Sensitive to	Resistant to
Penicillin	Erythromycin
Ampicillin	Aminoglycosides
Cephalosporins	Trimethoprim
Chloramphenicol	

Higher than normal dose rates of antibiotics are recommended in bacterial endocarditis, and the intravenous route is preferred initially.

It is important to treat concomitant problems, and care needs to be taken in geriatric patients when using drugs such as the aminoglycosides which may be nephrotoxic.

3. Dilated cardiomyopathy

Incidence

Dilated cardiomyopathy (DCM) usually occurs in young to middle age dogs (range 6 months to 14 years, mean 4–6 years) of giant breeds, however in the boxer the mean age at presentation is reported to be 8 years (Fox 1988) and so the condition is included in this chapter. In boxers more males are affected than females and there is greater prevalence in some breeding lines.

DCM affects mainly young to middle aged cats, and is often associated with taurine deficiency. Taurine deficiency has been identified as a cause of DCM in cats fed commercial petfoods that failed to maintain satisfactory plasma taurine concentrations. It is not considered further here.

Gross pathology

Severe dilatation of all chambers of the heart is characteristic of the condition in most breeds, but this is not true in the boxer. There is thinning of the ventricular walls (unless compensatory hypertrophy is present) and atrophy of papillary muscles and trabeculae. Focal endocardial fibrosis is present.

In boxers there is usually thickening of the atrioventricular valves (mitral, but sometimes the tricuspid or aortic valve).

Histopathology

Myocardial degeneration.

Aetiopathogenesis

The aetiology is unknown in most cases. Metabolic defects have been demonstrated in some species and carnitine-related problems in the myocardium have been reported in some dogs, including boxers with DCM.

Selenium deficiency has been implicated but not proven in some cases as have toxins, infective agents (viruses) and immunological factors.

Pathophysiology

Impaired ventricular contractility leads to reduced ejection volume, though compensatory mechanisms such as increased heart rate may maintain cardiac output for a short period. Reduced renal blood flow stimulates the renin–angiotensin–aldosterone–antidiuretic hormone (ADH) pathway causing sodium and water retention increasing preload and afterload. Increased sympathetic tone also increases preload, and results in peripheral vasoconstriction further reducing cardiac output. Congestive heart failure eventually develops.

Clinical findings

 (1) weakness
 (2) congestive heart failure
 (3) syncope
 (4) pale membranes, prolonged capillary refill times
 (5) ascites, hepatosplenomaegaly
 (6) mitral murmur
 (7) weight loss
 (8) arrhythmias (atrial fibrillation often – but not in boxers)
 (9) cardiomegaly on radiographs
(10) ECG changes.

About one-half of the boxers with DCM have no significant radiographic abnormalities present, and about one-third of boxers are asymptomatic.

ECG changes most typical for the boxer are ventricular premature complexes and paroxysmal ventricular tachycardia.

Endomyocardial biopsy has confirmed carnitine-deficiency in some boxers with DCM, and dietary supplementation may be beneficial.

Treatment

- inotropic agents
- diuretics
- vasodilators
- antiarrhythmic drugs
- dietary modification
- restricted exercise.

4. Neoplasia

In dogs haemangiosarcoma is the most common primary cardiac neoplasm and it usually affects the right atrium. They may also be secondary having spread from another site. The German shepherd dog may be predisposed to develop this type of tumour.

Heart base tumours (chemodectomas) are most commonly found in brachycephalic dogs such as the boxer and Boston terrier (6–14 years of age) and males may be affected more frequently. The tumours usually involve the aortic bodies lying at the base of the aorta and pulmonary artery. They are often small and slow growing, but can infiltrate locally. Ectopic thyroid or parathyroid tumours and lymphomas may also occur at this site.

In cats primary cardiac tumours are rare. Haemangiosarcoma and lymphosarcoma are the most common secondary metastatic neoplasms.

Clinical findings

Depending upon the structures invaded or compressed by the growing tumour mass a variety of clinical findings can be seen:

(1) dysrhythmias
(2) signs of congestive heart failure
(3) pericardial effusion (haemorrhage) with/without tamponade
(4) syncope
(5) weakness
(6) weight loss
(7) dyspnoea.

Diagnosis

Based on clinical findings, radiography, echocardiography.

Treatment

Although surgical excision may be possible in some cases, treatment is usually inadvisable as the prognosis is poor.

5. Feline hyperthyroidism

Incidence

Hyperthyroidism, or thyrotoxicosis is a common condition of older cats (6–20 years) with a reported incidence of 1/300 cats. There is no breed or sex predilection.

Gross pathology

Cats with hyperthyroidism are usually thin or emaciated. They have unilateral or bilateral enlargement of the thyroid glands.

Histopathology

Benign functional adenoma (adenomatous hyperplasia) of the thyroid gland. Thyroid carcinomas rarely cause hyperthyroidism in the cat.

Aetiopathogenesis

Unknown.

Pathophysiology

Cardiac changes in hyperthyroidism are due to the direct effects of increased thyroid hormone secretion on the heart, and increased adrenergic stimulation. These changes include increased heart rate, contractility, ejection fraction (at rest but not during exercise), pulse pressure and cardiac output.

Secondary hypertrophic cardiomyopathy may occur, or the condition may progress to congestive heart failure.

Clinical findings

The following are most frequently noted:

(1) weight loss
(2) polyphagia
(3) hyperactivity
(4) tachycardia
(5) polydipsia/polyuria
(6) cardiac murmur
(7) vomiting
(8) diarrhoea.

Enlargement of the thyroid gland(s) can usually be palpated and may be unilateral or bilateral. A chain of thyroid masses may extend down the neck and through the thoracic inlet.

On ECG sinus tachycardia and large R waves are seen in lead II (> 0.9 mV). Arrhythmias are also often present.

Chest radiographs reveal left-sided cardiac enlargement with other signs of congestive heart failure, e.g. pulmonary oedema and/or pleural effusion. Echocardiography demonstrates left ventricular dilatation, hypertrophy and increased contractility. These changes are reversible once the hyperthyroidism is corrected.

Radionuclide imaging is helpful to confirm whether both lobes of the thyroid are involved, to identify small adenomatous changes, to detect intrathoracic remnants and to identify metastases.

Laboratory findings

Elevated T4 concentrations and usually elevated T3 as well.

These cases also may have elevated alanine aminotransferase (ALT), aspartate aminotransferase (AST), serum alkaline phosphatase (SAP) and lactate dehydrogenase (LDH) concentrations. Hyperphosphataemia sometimes occurs.

Leukocytosis, eosinopenia and increased packed cell volume are commonly found.

Diagnosis

Clinical findings, elevated T4 concentrations, palpation of enlarged thyroid lobe(s).

Treatment

Primary objective is to create a euthyroid state:

(1) thyroidectomy – treatment of choice
(2) antithyroid drugs – carbimazole 10–15 mg daily in divided doses for 1–3 weeks
(3) radioactive iodine therapy.

Specific treatment for the secondary cardiac disease should only be given if needed:

(1) diuretics (frusemide 1 mg/kg, b.i.d. to t.i.d.) if oedema or pleural effusion is severe
(2) oral propranolol if tachydysrhythmias are severe at a dose of 2.5 mg b.i.d. to t.i.d. up to 6 kg body weight (for cats over 6 kg body weight give 5 mg b.i.d. to t.i.d.).

6. Cor pulmonale

Cor pulmonale is right heart disease secondary to pulmonary vascular or parenchymal disease. It is common in brachycephalic dogs with chronic airway obstruction due to stenosis of the nares, or collapse of the trachea or bronchi, or chronic bronchitis.

Aetiopathogenesis

Several causes have been described:

(1) Primary lung disease. In geriatric dogs the most common cause is chronic obstructive pulmonary disease (which includes bronchitis and emphysema).
(2) Pulmonary vascular obstruction due to heartworm, thromboembolism, or compression by neoplastic or other masses.
(3) Obesity restricting chest wall movement resulting in poor inspiration and hypoxaemia (Pickwickian-syndrome).
(4) Thoracic deformity such as pectus excavatum.

Pathophysiology

Pulmonary arterial hypertension leads to right-sided cardiac enlargement, with myocardial hypertrophy progressing to right ventricular failure.

Clinical findings

Onset may be acute or chronic. Severe cases may present with air hunger and abdominal breathing, cyanosis or sudden death; milder cases with anorexia, weakness, depression, wheezing, dyspnoea, panting, coughing, signs of right-sided congestive heart failure.

It is a diagnostic challenge to differentiate between a chronic cough caused by atrial compression or a mainstem bronchus, and a cough caused by chronic obstructive pulmonary disease, particularly in geriatric patients as both conditions frequently occur together. Nevertheless correct diagnosis is essential if treatment is to prove successful.

Auscultation may reveal abnormal lung sounds depending upon the amount of fluid secretion. Heart sounds may be normal, or there may be a split second sound, and sometimes there is a murmur caused by tricuspid insufficiency.

2.5 TREATMENT OF GERIATRIC HEART DISEASE

Rational treatment of cardiovascular disease depends upon accurate diagnosis of the type of heart disease present. Most forms of heart disease are progressive and treatment is aimed at controlling the signs of failure and delaying progression, it does not change the underlying pathology.

Left-sided heart failure

Left-sided heart failure causes increased pulmonary venous pressure and pulmonary oedema. The animal presents with pulmonary signs due to congestion, i.e. coughing, increased respiratory noise on auscultation, dyspnoea, orthopnoea, cyanosis. Excitation or exertion usually exacerbate the signs.

Left-sided heart failure is common in geriatric patients being caused by chronic valvular endocardiosis and cardiomyopathies which are both common, and myocarditis which is rare.

Right-sided heart failure

Results in congestion of abdominal organs causing hepatomegaly, splenomegaly, distended caudal vena cava and jugular veins, pericardial effusions and ascites or intrathoracic effusions. Peripheral oedema rarely occurs.

Tricuspid insufficiency, cor pulmonale and neoplasia of the right side of the heart are the geriatric diseases which would most likely cause right heart failure in the UK, but the pulmonary hypertension that occurs with left-sided heart failure may result eventually in right-sided failure as well. In enzootic areas heartworm can also cause right heart failure at any age.

Myocardial failure

Is characterised by the presence of a weak pulse, pallor, cold extremeties, with exercise intolerance and sometimes the development of prerenal azotaemia.

Staging heart failure

Four clinical stages of progressive heart failure have been defined by the New York Heart Association and these are useful when determining the most appropriate treatment regimen for individual cases (Table 2.3). Contrary to the conventional view of veterinary cardiologists, the author believes that sodium restriction and obesity control should be started as early as possible in the course of heart disease, i.e. during stage I.

Table 2.3 Usual staging of chronic left-sided heart failure due to endocardiosis.

Stage	Definition	Treatment
I	Murmur present (Grade I–II) but no fatigue, dyspnoea or coughing	No therapy usually advised – but dietary intake of sodium should be controlled, and obesity corrected
II	Dog comfortable at rest but cough present, may have delayed return to normal heart rate following exercise, and may have respiratory sounds	Exercise should be restricted Dietary control over sodium intake and excessive body weight Xanthine derivatives or diuretics
III	Laboured respiration and poor exercise tolerance, in addition to coughing	Minimise exercise Digitalisation may be necessary and vosodilators may be helpful
IV	Decompensated congestive heart failure with dyspnoea, orthopnoea and coughing even at rest	Cage rest, diuresis and sedation if excitable Digitalisation if tachycardia or cardiomyopathy Vasodilator therapy Antidysrhythmic drugs if necessary

DIET

Energy

At the time of presentation many animals with heart disease will exhibit cardiac cachexia and several mechanisms for this have been proposed:

(1) Anorexia – due to the disease itself but also commonly associated with some therapeutic agents.
(2) Malabsorption – due to compromised gastrointestinal function.
(3) Peripheral tissue deterioration due to underperfusion.
(4) Hypermetabolism of respiratory and cardiac tissues.
(5) Generalised hypermetabolism due to fever, sepsis or stress. The chronic sympathetic stimulation which is a normal compensatory mechanism in response to falling cardiac output will induce a catabolic state in the patient and may lead to peripheral insulin resistance.

Cardiac patients have high energy requirements and need an increased energy intake. Fat provides 2.25 times as much energy per gram as either protein or carbohydrate, hence a high-fat diet is indicated. A high fat diet is also beneficial because the amount of food that an animal with heart disease needs to consume to meet its requirements is reduced, and fat in a ration increases its palatability. Clinical diseases associated with excessive fat consumption that are common in man (e.g. severe coronary artery disease and atherosclerosis) are fortunately rare in old cats and dogs.

For debilitated cases special feeding techniques may need to be employed including force feeding or tube feeding.

Salt intake

Dogs with subclinical as well as clinical heart disease have impaired sodium regulation (Hamlin *et al.* 1967). Dogs with progressive valvular endo-cardiosis may have sodium retention during the prodromal (or compensated) phase of the disease. This is a reasonable conclusion because one of the body's compensatory mechanisms in the presence of reducing cardiac output is sodium and water retention by activation of the renin–angiotensin–aldosterone–ADH pathway and aldosterone concentrations have been found to be increased in dogs with spontaneous heart failure.

Sodium retention increases preload on the heart and may lead to hypertension, oedema and ascites.

Plasma sodium concentrations may also be affected by two situations commonly found in geriatrics:

(1) Reduced daily water intake – the thirst centre is reported to be less sensitive to hyperosmolarity in older animals.
(2) Renal insufficiency – leads to sodium retention.

Contrary to popular belief, there is no documented evidence that dogs resist change from a high salt to a low salt diet. In one practice survey, only one client in ten reported any difficulty in getting their dog to accept a very low salt diet, and that was not due to poor palatability (Sauvage J. 1990, personal communication).

If changing from a high salt diet to a low salt diet is going to be a problem, it is likely to be so in:

(1) older dogs with an acquired taste for high salt diets which has been reinforced over many years; and
(2) a dog which is inappetent due to the onset of congestive heart failure.

There is no evidence that high salt intake is beneficial to an animal with heart disease.

For these reasons the author believes that sodium intake should be reduced *as early as possible* in the progression of heart disease, i.e. during Stage 1.

The sodium contents of 'low sodium' diets available in the UK are listed in Table 2.4. All of these diets actually exceed the minimum daily sodium requirement, but compared with other available foods they reduce excessive sodium intake. Reducing sodium intake reduces preload on the heart.

Table 2.4 Sodium content of special diets available for the management of cardiac disease in cats and dogs.

Diet	Sodium content %	Energy density (kcal/100 gm)
Hill's Prescription Diet Canine h/d (canned)	0.023 (as fed) 0.08 (dry matter basis)	143 (as fed) 514 (dry matter basis)
Hill's Prescription Diet Canine h/d (dry)	0.05% (as fed) 0.05% (dry matter)	429 (as fed) 464 (dry matter)
Hill's Presciption Diet Feline h/d (canned)	0.08% (as fed) 0.28% (dry matter)	127 (as fed) 439 (dry matter)
Pedigree Canine Low Sodium Diet (canned)	0.03 (as fed) 0.10 (dry matter)	155 (as fed)

The daily sodium intake is dependent upon the energy density of the food as well as the amount of sodium in the diet. The higher the energy density the less food is needed, so a high energy, low salt diet is recommended.

When changing from a relatively high salt diet, it is best to introduce the new food gradually over a period of 10–14 days, and tit-bits and snacks must be avoided as these are often high in salt content.

'Low salt' diets should not be given to animals that have hyponatraemia (rare), chronic debilitation or chronic diarrhoea.

Other minerals

Long-term diuretic therapy may lead to significant urinary losses of magnesium, iron and zinc, and sometimes potassium. Hypokalaemia may potentiate the toxic effects of digitalis glycosides.

Protein

Hypoproteinaemia is sometimes associated with heart failure due to:

- malabsorption
- removal of fluid accumulations, e.g. ascites.

Dietary recommendations

Compared with a maintenance ration the basic profile of a diet for a geriatric animal with heart disease should be:

- low sodium
- high energy density
- increased water soluble vitamins*
- increased trace elements*
- increased potassium†
- high palatability
- high digestibility
- high biological value ingredients.
  * In the presence of increased diuresis
  † Care if using potassium-sparing diuretics.

  Avoid:

- high sodium intake (particularly snacks/tit-bits)
- excessive potassium intake (may cause hyperkalaemia)
- obesity
- too rapid a weight-loss programme (> 3% body weight loss/week for dogs; > 1% body weight loss/week for cats)
- poorly digestible/poor quality raw ingredients

- low biological value ingredients
- any nutritional excess, deficiency or imbalance.

Some animals will have hypoproteinaemia, in which case adequate high biological value protein intake must be maintained, but at the same time excessive protein should be avoided to minimise metabolic stress on liver and kidney particularly if there is evidence of reduced function. Protein intake needs to be adjusted to suit each individual.

DRUGS

Diuretics
Frusemide and the thiazide diuretics induce water loss by their saluretic action, so concomitant reduction of dietary salt intake is logical and may reduce the dose of diuretic needed. Conversely, high salt intake in patients which have sodium retention may increase the dose of diuretic needed.

Diuretics are indicated when the signs of congestion, oedema, ascites or volume overload cannot be controlled by reduced salt intake alone.

Typically dogs in Stages III and IV of heart failure will benefit from diuretics, but some individuals in Stage II may also require low dose diuretic administration.

Diuretics given in heart failure will reduce circulating blood volume (hypovolaemia) thereby reducing preload effects on the heart, and loop diuretics may cause peripheral vasodilation which also reduces cardiac workload. However, the reduced renal blood flow which also results may be undesirable as it decreases glomerular filtration rate and renal function, and may precipitate acute renal failure.

Other undesirable effects of diuretic use include hypokalaemia, hyponatraemia, hypocalcaemia and hypomagnesaemia. Relative overdosage may cause dehydration and if extracellular fluid is lost without bicarbonate loss, metabolic alkalosis. Some authors advocate routine monitoring of body weight, creatinine, acid–base balance and serum electrolytes (particularly potassium) during diuretic therapy.

Hypokalaemia enhances cardiac glycoside toxicity, may cause cardiac dysrhythmias and impairs carbohydrate metabolism.

Hypomagnesaemia potentiates the cardiac effects of hypokalaemia.

Dietary potassium supplementation with salt substitute (KCl) may be helpful in avoiding hypokalaemia, and the use of potassium sparing diuretics such as spironolactone, amiloride or triamterene in conjunction with more potent diuretics such as frusemide, will also help reduce the chances of the development of hypokalaemia, but these drugs should not be used in the presence of other age-related conditions which might predispose to hyperkalaemia such as renal failure or diabetes mellitus. They should also not be used in the presence of metabolic acidosis or alongside therapy with beta-blockers or angiotensin-converting enzyme (ACE) inhibitors (e.g. captopril).

To avoid iatrogenic hyperkalaemia, potassium supplementation should not be given at the same time as the potassium-sparing diuretics.

The efficacy of diuretics may be reduced in the presence of hypoproteinaemia (as they are protein-bound), proteinuria or impaired renal function.

Osmotic diuretics such as mannitol are contraindicated in heart disease, as they may cause cardiac overload.

Hydrochlorothiazide

Thiazide diuretic indicated for oedema associated with cardiac failure.

Dose
Dogs and cats: 1–2 mg/kg daily, orally.
                  12–25 mg, daily, i.m.

Frusemide

Loop diuretic indicated for oedema associated with cardiac failure.

Contraindications
Renal impairment with anuria.

Side-effects
May cause hypokalaemia if used long term. May potentiate toxicity of the cardiac glycosides.

Dose
Dogs and cats   5 mg/kg, 1–2 times daily, orally.
                 2.5–5 mg/kg, 1–2 times daily, i.v. or i.m.

Spironolactone, amiloride hydrochloride and triamterene

Potassium sparing diuretics which also reduce magnesium loss. Indicated for oedema associated with cardiac failure.

Contraindications
Concurrent potassium supplements and beta-blockers, renal impairment, metabolic acidosis, diabetes mellitus.

Dose
Spironolactone
Dogs and cats   1–2 mg/kg daily, orally.

Amiloride hydrochloride
Dogs and cats   1–2 mg/kg daily, orally.

Triamterene
Dogs and cats   0.5–3 mg/kg daily, orally.

Vasodilators
These drugs act primarily on the peripheral vasculature and reduce the workload on the heart. Some vasodilators, e.g. nitrates, cause venodilation, reducing venous return to the heart, and thereby decreasing systemic and pulmonary venous pressures (preload). Others, e.g. hydralazine, cause arteriodilation thus reducing afterload on the left ventricle. Some vasodilators, e.g. prazosin, nitroprusside and the angiotensin-converting enzyme (ACE) inhibitors (e.g. enalapril and captopril) have effects on preload and afterload.

Conventional vasodilators such as hydralazine and isosorbide dinitrate stimulate the sympathetic system and the renin–angiotensin–aldosterone–ADH system resulting in sodium and water retention, which may be detrimental to some patients. Therefore they are probably best used in combination with cardiac glycosides and diuretics.

Concurrent treatment with ACE inhibitors (e.g. enalapril) offers a good therapeutic approach to clinical cases not responding to diuretics and digoxin therapy alone. Marked hypotension can be a problem following the initial oral dose of an ACE inhibitor particularly in patients on diuretics or on a low salt diet, and patients are best hospitalised during the introduction of ACE inhibitors. Any drug that induces hypotension may precipitate prerenal azotaemia and acute renal failure in at-risk patients, and ACE inhibitors are contraindicated in the presence of renal impairment. In old animals renal function should be monitored closely before, and for at least a week after the use of these drugs, and diuretic doses should be reduced when they are administered at the same time.

Benazepril

An angiotensin-converting enzyme (ACE) inhibitor. Indicated for the treatment of heart failure in dogs.

Contraindications
Aortic stenosis. May interact with the drug spironolactone. It is claimed that this drug is less likely to accumulate in the presence of renal impairment because it is excreted in bile.

Side-effects
Signs of hypotension such as tiredness, may occur.

Dose
Dogs   0.25–0.5 mg/kg body weight, daily.

Captopril

An angiotensin-converting enzyme (ACE) inhibitor. Indicated for congestive heart failure.

Contraindications
Renal impairment.

Side-effects
Hypotension, renal failure, gastrointestinal disorders, anorexia.

Dose
Start with low doses due to hypotensive effects.

Dogs   0.25–2 mg/kg, t.i.d. orally.

Cats   4–6 mg, t.i.d. orally.

Enalapril maleate

Indicated for the treatment of congestive heart failure in dogs caused by mitral regurgitation or dilated cardiomyopathy as an adjunctive therapy with diuretics. To improve exercise tolerance and increase survival in dogs with moderate or several congestive heart failure.

Side-effects
Hypotension, azotaemia, lethargy, drowsiness, inco-ordination. Hyperkalaemia.

Dose
Dogs   0.5 mg/kg once daily for 2 weeks increasing to a maximum dose of 0.5 mg/kg b.i.d. if necessary.

Cats   Contraindicated.

Hydralazine

Indicated for mitral regurgitation and left-sided heart failure.

Side-effects
Tachycardia, hypotension, gastrointestinal disorders, depression, anorexia.

Dose
Dogs   0.5–3 mg/kg b.i.d.

Cats   2.5 mg b.i.d.

Glyceryl trinitrate

Indicated for pulmonary oedema secondary to heart failure. **Warning: Always wear gloves when handling preparation.**

Contraindications
Cardiogenic shock.

Side-effects
Hypotension.

Dose
Dogs and cats   Topical administration 0.5–2 centimetres of a 2% ointment to inaccessible part of skin, e.g. pinna of ear.

Prazosin hydrochloride

Indicated for congestive heart failure. **Warning: For animals over 5 kg body weight only.**

Side-effects
Hypotension.

Dose
Dogs   5–15 kg body weight 1 mg 2–3 times daily.
Over 15 kg 2 mg 2–3 times daily.

Sodium nitroprusside

Indicated for severe congestive heart failure.

Side-effects
Hypotension.

Dose
Intravenous 1 µg/kg per minute to maintain arterial BP over 70 mmHG.

Cardiac glycosides

The cardiac glycosides are used for their positive inotropic effects by enhancing calcium influx into myocardial cells increasing the force of contraction of the myocardium, and also for their negative chronotropic effect in reducing the rate of myocardial contraction. In elderly people and horses, the main indication for cardiac glycosides is for heart failure in the presence of atrial fibrillation. In cats and dogs the main indication is for supraventricular arrhythmias, or for myocardial failure (i.e. congestive heart failure).

Digoxin is cleared mainly via glomerular filtration in the kidney (half-life 20–35 hours) whereas digitoxin is cleared via the liver (half-life 8–12 hours) thus concomitant organ disease should be considered and screened out *before* their administration.

In humans digoxin clearance in the elderly is equivalent to the creatinine clearance and its half-life is prolonged in elderly patients. The same is probably true in geriatric dogs and cats, thus sensitivity to digoxin toxicity may be greater in older animals. It has been suggested that the dose of digoxin should be halved if azotaemia is present but a better approach would be to give digitoxin instead.

Digitoxin can be cleared by the liver even in the presence of liver disease.

Both digoxin and digitoxin have a narrow therapeutic margin and there are many factors that may increase the sensitivity of a patient to toxic side-effects including: age, hypokalaemia, hypomagnesaemia, hypercalcaemia, acidosis, calcium channel blockers, antibiotics, renal failure, hypothyroidism.

Special care is needed in the administration of these drugs to geriatric patients, and screening for subclinical conditions which might enhance toxic side-effects or alter efficacy is mandatory.

The value of monitoring serum digoxin concentrations has been questioned because of overlap in digoxin concentrations seen in groups of patients with and without toxic side-effects, and also because false elevations may be seen in sera from patients with chronic renal failure or liver disease.

Contraindications
Renal impairment, sinus or AV node disease (arrhythmias).

Digoxin

Dose
Dogs   10 µg/kg b.i.d. (max 750 µg).

Cats   7–15 µg/kg every other day.

The digoxin elixir is more readily absorbed from the gastrointestinal tract than tablets, hence the dose should be reduced.

Digitoxin

Dose
Dogs only   40–100 µ/kg daily in 3 divided doses.

Side-effects:
Depression, anorexia, vomiting, diarrhoea, bradycardia (sino-atrial block), arrhythmias, acute renal failure.

Digitalis intoxication is common in practice. Withdraw treatment for 2–3 days, or longer if the toxicity is severe. Give supportive treatment, e.g. fluids and potassium supplementation. Once stabilised reintroduce drug at 50–75% original dose. If necessary use an alternative inotrope such as dobutamine.

Sympathomimetic drugs

Dobutamine hydrochloride

A synthetic catecholamine (sympathomimetic) which acts by stimulating β- and α-adrenergic activity and increases myocardial contractility. Indicated for cardiogenic shock, bradycardia, dilated cardiomyopathy, congestive heart failure.

Side-effects
Tachycardia – should monitor ECG.

Dose

Dogs   2–7 µg/kg per minute i.v. infusion for up to 3 days.

Cats   4 µg/kg per minute by i.v. infusion.

Adrenaline

A sympathomimetic drug which acts on both α- and β-receptors increasing heart rate and contractility, and causing peripheral vasodilation or vaso-constriction.

Indicated for cardiac arrest.

Dose*

Dogs and cats   2–5 µg/kg, intracardiac
                 0.5–10 µg/kg, i.v.

*Use 1 in 10 000 dilution

Antimuscarinic drugs

Atropine sulphate

An antimuscarinic drug indicated for bradycardia, AV block, sino-atrial arrest.

Contraindications

Glaucoma.

Side-effects

Tachycardia, urinary retention, constipation, pupillary dilatation.

Dose

Dogs and cats   10–20 µg/kg, i.m. or i.v.
                 30–40 µg/kg, s.c.

Antiarrhythmics

These drugs are used to regulate cardiac rate or rhythm. See also cardiac glycosides, sympathomimetics and atropine.

Class IA antiarrhythmics

Quinidine sulphate

This slows conduction, depresses inotropism and causes arteriolar dila-tation by blocking α-receptors. It is sometimes used to treat atrial, junctional and ventricular premature complexes and ventricular tachycardia in the dog. Occasionally it is used for atrial fibrillation.

Contraindications
Hepatic impairment.

Dose
Dogs   4–16 mg/kg, 3–4 times daily

Route of excretion: hepatic

Quinidine (and verapamil) reduce renal excretion and can increase digoxin concentrations. Quinidine also displaces digoxin from muscle binding sites increasing serum levels, therefore use of this drug is contra-indicated in digoxin toxicity.

Increased plasma quinidine concentrations may be caused by con-current use of acetazolamide, antacids; cimetidine; diuretics (hypokalae-mia), and the concurrent use of muscle relaxants, neostigmine or warfarin are not advised.

Procainamide hydrochloride

The drug of choice to treat ventricular premature complexes and ven-tricular tachycardia in the dog.

Contraindications
Atrial fibrillation, renal impairment, heart blocks.

Side-effects
Gastrointestinal disturbances.

Dose
Dogs   8–20 mg/kg, 3–4 times daily, orally.
8–20 mg/kg 4 times daily, i.m.
2–15 mg/kg over 20 min, then constant infusion at 10–40 µg/ kg per min, i.v.

N.B. These drugs may cause hypotension and anticholinergic effects.

Class IB antiarrhythmics
Lignocaine and *phenytoin*. These drugs decrease cardiac tissue auto-maticity and are useful in the treatment of ventricular tachycardia in the dog. Phenytoin is particularly useful in the management of tachycardias associated with digitalis toxicity.

Lignocaine

Lignocaine is not effective in the presence of hypokalaemia associated with loop thiazide diuretics. Toxicity may be enhanced by cimetidine, and if used simultaneously with beta-blockers there is increased risk of myocardial depression and bradycardia.

Contraindications
Atrial fibrillation or flutter.

Dose

Dogs   2 mg/kg i.v. bolus followed by constant i.v. infusion at 50 µg/kg per min.

Cats   250–500 µg i.v. bolus followed by constant i.v. infusion at 20 µg/kg per min. (N.B. Cats are very sensitive to neuroexcitatory side-effects).

Dose should be reduced in the presence of congestive heart failure.

Route of excretion: hepatic. Propranolol and cimetidine both decrease hepatic blood flow and could predispose to toxicity if used simultaneously.

Phenytoin

Dose
Dogs only   35–50 mg/kg, orally, t.i.d.

Class II antiarrhythmics
Beta-blockers which inhibit sympathetic activity. They decrease SA node rate and prolong AV node conduction.

Propranolol hydrochloride

Indicated for supraventricular tachycardia, hypertrophic cardiomyopathy, hyperthyroidism (cats), atrial and ventricular premature dysrhythmias.

Contraindications
Hepatic impairment, respiratory disease particularly involving the small airways, sick sinus syndrome, AV block, cardiac output failure.

Side-effects
Bronchospasm, myocardial depression, bradycardia, hypotension.

Hypotension may lead to pre-renal azotaemia, particularly if the drug is administered concomitantly with a diuretic.

The negative inotropic side-effects may exacerbate signs of congestive heart failure.

Dose

Dogs   100 μg/kg t.i.d. increasing over 3–5 days up to 1 mg/kg t.i.d. (as needed).

Cats   2.5 mg t.i.d. increasing over 3–5 days up to 10 mg t.i.d. (as needed).

Atenolol

Indicated for supraventricular arrhythmias.

For side-effects and contraindications see propranolol.

Dose

Dogs   20–100 mg t.i.d.

Timolol maleate

Indicated for supraventricular arrhythmias.

For side-effects and contraindications see propranolol.

Dose

Dogs   0.5–5 mg t.i.d.

Class IV antiarrhythmics

Calcium channel blockers, causing arterial and venous dilation.

Drugs of choice for severe supraventricular tachyarrhythmias.

They cause coronary artery dilatation and hypotension due to peripheral vasodilation. They have a negative inotropic effect.

Diltiazem hydrochloride

Indicated for the treatment of supraventricular tachyarrhythmias.

Side-effects

Hypotension, bradycardia.

Dose

Dogs   0.5–1.25 mg/kg 3–4 times daily.

Cats   1.5–2 mg/kg 2–3 times daily.

Verapamil hydrochloride

Indicated for supraventricular tachyarrhythmias

Side-effects

Hypotension, bradycardia, myocardial depression.
    Care needed in congestive heart failure cases.

Dose

Dogs   1–5 mg/kg, t.i.d., orally.
        50–150 µg/kg i.v. to effect.

REFERENCES AND FURTHER READING

Detweiler, D.K. & Patterson, D.F. (1965) The prevalence and types of cardio-vascular disease in dogs. *Annals of the New York Academy of Science*, **127**, 481–516.

Detweiler, D.K. *et al.* (1968) The natural history of acquired cardiac disability of the dog. *Annals of the New York Academy of Science*, **147**, 318–29.

Ettinger, S.J. & Suter, P.F. (1970) *Canine Cardiology*. W.B. Saunders, Philadelphia.

Fox, P.R. (1988) *Canine and Feline Cardiology*. Churchill-Livingstone, Edinburgh.

Hamlin, R.L., Smith, C.R. & Ross, J.N. (1967) Detection and quantitation of subclinical heart failure in dogs. *Journal of the American Veterinary Medical Association*, **150**(12), 1513–15.

Jonsson, L. (1972) Coronary arterial lesions and myocardial infarcts in the dog. *Acta Veterinaria Scandinavica Supplement*, **38**, 7–73.

Maher, E.R. & Rush, J.E. (1990) Cardiovascular changes in the geriatric dog. *Compendium on Continuing Education – Special Focus Canine Geriatrics*, **12**(7), 921–31.

Mosier, J.E. (1987) How aging affects body systems of the dog. In: *Geriatric Medicine: Contemporary Clinical and Practice Management Approaches*. p. 3. Veterinary Medicine Publishing Company, Topeka, Kansas.

Valtonen, M.H. (1972) Cardiovascular disease and nephritis in dogs. *Journal of Small Animal Practice*, **13**, 687–97.

Whitney, J.C. (1974) Observations on the effect of age on the severity of heart valve lesions in the dog. *Journal of Small Animal Practice*, **15**, 511–22.

Yin, F.C., Spurgeon, H.A., Greene, H.L. *et al.* (1979) Age associated decrease in heart rate response to isoproterenol in dogs. *Mechanisms of Ageing and Development*, **10**, 17–25.

Yin, F.C., Weisfeldt, M.L. & Milnor, W.R. (1981) Role of aortic input impedance in the decreased cardiovascular response to exercise with aging in dogs. *Journal of Clinical Investigation*, **68**, 28–38.

Chapter 3
THE NERVOUS SYSTEM

KEY POINTS

(1) Age-related changes in the central and peripheral nervous systems (CNS and PNS) are responsible for many of the physiological and behavioural changes commonly associated with advancing age and senility.

(2) Many of the age-related degenerative CNS changes reported to occur in humans are believed by veterinary neurologists to occur in dogs and cats but they have been poorly documented.

(3) In decision making about treatment and prognosis it is important to relate observed neurological changes to the site of the underlying lesion. For example, it is important to differentiate upper motor neuron deficits from lower motor neuron deficits in patients with locomotor disease.

(4) The onset of seizures in old animals should promote a search for extracranial causes (e.g. hepatic disease) and for structural lesions in the CNS (e.g. brain tumours).

(5) Old patients requiring anticonvulsant therapy for seizures should be screened for liver disease and should be monitored for early detection of hepatotoxicity.

(6) Neuroendocrine disorders are probably much more common in old animals than is currently recognised clinically.

(7) The process of ageing may be a manifestation of a failure to regulate neuroendocrine function *or* ageing may be dependent upon neuroendocrine regulation running in parallel with other temporal factors ... the so-called genetic 'programming', 'clock' or 'pacemaker' theory.

(8) Regular exercise is an important stimulator of neuroendocrine function and should be maintained throughout old age.

3.1 INTRODUCTION

Age-related changes in the CNS or PNS may result in decreased or increased activity of neural tissue with corresponding signs of altered neurological or neuroendocrine function. A skilled clinician can determine the site of the changes from the neurological signs exhibited by an animal.

Reduced protein synthesis within cells is one of the main causes of age-related declines in tissue function and some authors believe that modification of neuroendocrine function offers the best prospect for delaying and reversing ageing changes (Meites 1993).

Modification of neuroendocrine function is probably one of the mechanisms by which calorie-restricted diets slow down ageing changes in body tissues, inhibit the development of disease and neoplasia, and significantly prolong the lifespan of rats and mice. Calorie-restricted diets decrease hormone secretion (in particular growth hormone and insulin-like growth factor 1) and also alter hormone receptor sensitivity, reduce whole-body metabolism (though basal metabolic rate per unit lean body mass remains the same) and lower gene expression.

As further support of this hypothesis the administration of hormones, thymic peptides and some drugs can improve declining immune function thus improving resistance to infections, neoplasia and autoimmune disorders.

In old dogs the administration of clonidine (an α 2-adrenergic agonist) increases the pulsatile secretion of growth hormone – returning it to a young dog type of pattern. Furthermore administration of clonidine with growth hormone releasing hormone for 10 days significantly increases both the peak concentration and total amount of growth hormone released. A rapid radio-immunoassay for growth hormone in the dog has been described (Cocola *et al.* 1976).

Maladaptive responses of the neuroendocrine system to stressful stimuli (particularly in the hypothalamic–pituitary–adrenocortical system) are thought to accelerate the ageing process and reduce longevity. One study in rats suggests that longevity is inversely related to hyperactivity to stress and that this is genotype dependent. Basal cortisol levels have been reported to be increased in dogs and to be related to cognitive dysfunction associated with ageing.

During ageing, humans, rats and dogs have been shown to have hypercortisolaemia and diffuse Alzheimer's-like brain lesions (extracellular β-A4-amyloid deposits and intracellular fibrillar structures (TAU-protein) called neurofibrillary tangles) and neuronal decay have been reported to occur in dog brains (Cummings *et al.* 1993; Morys 1994). Recently a direct correlation has been demonstrated between behaviour changes as determined by cognitive tests and the severity of these pathological changes in beagles and these workers have suggested that cushingoid dogs might be a useful model for the study of Alzheimer's disease in humans (Ruehl, W.W. 1995, personal communication).

Free radical damage may play a part in the age-related changes in catecholamine neurones in the hypothalamus and in the neurotransmission of catecholamines, acetylcholine and peptide co-transmitters. Changes in receptor-site numbers or sensitivity may decrease secretion from cells which are otherwise still capable of manufacturing hormones.

3.2 AGE-RELATED TISSUE CHANGES

Central nervous system

In most organs ageing results in reduced cell division and replacement of active cells with connective tissue, however in the brain there is little connective tissue and postmitotic neuronal death results in a proliferation of active glial elements.

With advancing age the CNS may undergo morphological and chemical changes (see Tables 3.1 and 3.2).

Table 3.1 Morphological changes that may been seen in the CNS with advancing age.

Reduced brain mass
Reduced number of neurones
Enlargement of the ventricles
Increased lipofuscin deposition in neurones
Leptomeningeal thickening
Reduced number (denudation) of dendritic spines
Astrocyte hypertrophy (gliosis)
Argyrophilic (senile) plaque formation
Corpora amylacea formation
Perivascular haemorrhage is reported to be common in very old dogs

Peripheral nervous system

Morphological changes

Segmental demyelination and wallerian-type degeneration have been described to occur with advancing age in humans, but the changes are usually mild. Slowing of peripheral and central nerve conduction has also been demonstrated in elderly people.

Peripheral neuropathies may develop secondary to metabolic diseases

Table 3.2 Chemical changes that may occur in the CNS with advancing age.

Increased water content in the brain.

Neurotransmitter enzyme concentrations may change with age.
In the monoaminergic system there are increased levels of monoamine oxidase and decreased levels of noradrenaline, dopamine and serotonin (5-HT).

Neurotransmitter receptors may change in number with age, for example D2 dopamine receptors reduce in number in rodents and humans, whereas the D1 dopamine receptors increase in number. Serotonin receptors S1 and S2 both decrease in numbers with age.

In the cholinergic system the presynaptic marker acetylcholinesterase is reported to increase in concentration with age whereas choline acetyltransferase decreases. There is a decrease in the number of muscarinic receptors. Neuropeptide neurotransmitters show variable age-related changes in concentrations in different regions of the brain.

Vascular disease such as arteriocapillary fibrosis or endothelial proliferation may reduce blood flow to the brain and so reduce oxygen transport and nutrient supply to the nerve cells, resulting in hypoxia and accumulation of intracellular waste products leading to functional decline with or without neuronal loss.

such as diabetes mellitus. In the cat diabetic neuropathy is associated with distal axonal degeneration and affected animals show hind limb paresis with distal muscle atrophy and hyporeflexia.

3.3   FUNCTIONAL CHANGES

There are many functional changes that can occur with advancing age:

Central nervous system

Impaired neurotransmission results from the decreased production of neurotransmitters and reduced breakdown of those that are produced.

Reduced serotonin levels increase sleeping time and may cause neuromuscular disorders and depression. Depletion of noradrenaline in the brain is also associated with depression.

Hypoxia leads to short-term memory loss, but not a loss of long-term memory. Oxygen supplementation can reverse this memory loss.

Signs of senility are frequently recognised in older animals and are probably associated with ageing changes in the nervous system but the precise cause–effect relationships have been poorly documented (see Table 3.3).

Regular exercise improves many bodily functions probably through its effects on the neuroendocrine system by increasing the secretion of

Table 3.3 Signs of senility frequently recognised in old cats and dogs.

Reduced mental alertness
Short-term memory loss
Reduced learning ability
Poor concentration – reduced attention span
Poor motor co-ordination
Delayed response to stimuli with slowed or decreased reflex responses
Loss of house training
Failure to recognise familiar surroundings/companions
Personality and other behavioural changes
Increased sleeping time

growth hormone and reducing the secretion of adrenocorticotrophic hormone (ACTH) and glucocorticoids.

Peripheral nervous system

With advancing age reduced function may occur in both the sympathetic and parasympathetic parts of the peripheral nervous system. Changes may be presynaptic, synaptic or postsynaptic resulting in impaired transmission of impulses to and from the CNS. This may produce abnormal neurological and neuromuscular function leading to sluggish reflexes, reduced pain response, impaired proprioception and difficulty with locomotion. The animal may be less able to respond to sudden stresses placed on it because of impaired ability to maintain homeostasis through neuroendocrine control mechanisms.

Inexperienced clinicians may find it difficult to differentiate between proprioceptive deficits and muscular weakness in older animals.

Treatment

Recently two drugs – propentofylline (Vivitonin, Hoechst) and nicergoline (Fitergol, Rhone Merieux) – have been granted veterinary product licences based upon their ability to improve the signs associated with ageing in dogs such as lethargy and dullness. They both have numerous pharmaceutical actions on the body but their main mechanism of action is thought to be an increase in blood supply to the brain resulting in improved neurological functions.

Propentofylline

Is indicated for the treatment of lethargy and dullness in old dogs.

Dose

12.5–100 mg b.i.d. depending upon body weight.

Nicergoline

Is an α-adrenoreceptor antagonist and is indicated in the treatment of age-related lethargy and dullness in dogs.

Dose

0.25–0.5 mg/kg daily.

3.4   NEUROLOGICAL DISEASES OF OLD AGE

CHRONIC 'OLD DOG' ENCEPHALITIS

Canine distemper is most prevalent in young dogs, but chronic 'old dog' encephalitis is the neurological manifestation of canine distemper virus (CDV) infection that is seen in adult dogs which have survived the acute infection. Dogs developing this condition are usually over 6 years of age and have serological evidence of systemic immunity.

The neurological signs (see Table 3.4) may occur without previous evidence of systemic disease and are usually progressive and irreversible (Greene and Appel 1990; Skerritt 1989). The involuntary muscle twitching (myoclonus) is typical of CDV infection.

Table 3.4 Neurological signs seen in the 'old dog encephalitis' form of canine distemper.

Hyperaesthesia
Cervical pain
Seizures
Cerebellar and vestibular signs
Visual deficits
Behavioural changes
Head-pressing
Circling
Paraparesis or tetraparesis
Ataxia
Myoclonus

CSF examination for increased protein and increased lymphocyte count may be helpful in diagnosing dogs exhibiting neurological signs.

Histologically there is perivascular lymphoplasmacytic infiltration in areas of demyelination and neuronal degeneration which may progress to sclerosing panencephalitis in more chronic cases. Canine distemper virus inclusion bodies are present in epithelial and other cells but their significance is not clear (Greene & Appel 1990).

Distemper can occur after stress, during concurrent illness or in immunesuppressed vaccinated dogs. Although vaccination with modified live CDV may confer long-term active immunity to some individuals, most manufacturers recommend booster vaccinations at 1–2 year intervals to ensure adequate ongoing protection.

The long-term prognosis is poor for most cases and, although some authors advocate a period of 1–2 weeks supportive therapy, euthanasia is usually the eventual outcome.

SEIZURES

Seizures can begin at any age and if they occur at a frequency greater than once every 6 weeks, or if the animal has clusters of seizures more than once every 8 weeks, anticonvulsant therapy is indicated.

The onset of seizures in old animals should prompt a search for an extracranial cause (e.g. hepatic disease) or an intracranial structural lesion (e.g. brain tumour).

Phenobarbitone and primidone are the drugs of choice for managing seizures in dogs, and phenobarbitone and diazepam for cats.

In 20–25% of dogs seizures are reported to be refractory to treatment with phenobarbitone and 40% and 48% of cases are refractory to primidone. Similar results have been reported for cats (Schwartz-Porsche 1992).

The most common cause of failure in treatment is inadequate dosage either by the clinician or due to owner non-compliance. The therapeutic range of serum concentration of phenobarbitone in the dog is 20–40 µg/ml and for the cat 10–30 µg/ml. The recommended dose rate is 1.5–5.0 mg/kg body weight but if adequate serum concentrations are achieved but seizure control does not occur even higher doses are recommended by some authors. Intervals between doses should be less than the half-life of the drug in the body to minimise fluctuations in serum concentrations.

The serum concentration of a drug is determined not only by dose but also by its bioavailability, metabolism and elimination. In older animals the objective should be to reduce the dose to the minimum needed to maintain serum concentrations within the recognised therapeutic range.

The recommended dose of anticonvulsants varies from one author/reference to another. During the initial treatment of refractory seizures the more rapidly the therapeutic dose is reached the greater the success so a high initial loading dose of phenobarbitone may be beneficial particularly for the most difficult seizures to control in dogs (clusters of generalized tonic-clonic seizures (GTCS)) and cats (complex focal seizures). For phenobarbitone a gradually increasing dose rate of up to 10–15 mg/kg body weight orally has been used for these cases (Schwartz-Porsche 1992).

Care is needed when using anticonvulsants in old animals – particularly if high doses are needed. The patient should be screened for evidence of impaired liver function and should be carefully monitored to ensure early detection of hepatotoxicity.

Primidone is not recommended at high dose rates for out-patients because it causes sedation. It is recommended to be given at 25 mg/kg body weight twice daily orally for both cats and dogs, though some authors advise administration at least three times daily.

Diazepam is the drug of choice for the initial control of status epilepticus in cats and dogs at a dose rate of 5–50 mg given i.v. in 5–10 mg doses followed by slow intravenous infusion at 2–5 mg/h in 5% glucose intravenous fluid. Orally diazepam is only 2–3% bioavailable but a dose of 0.5–2.0 mg/kg t.t.d. has been recommended for cats.

Potassium bromide and mephenytoin have been used successfully as adjuvants to conventional treatment but combination therapy should only be tried if drugs by themselves have proved to be unsuccessful. See Schwartz-Porsche 1992 for a review of adjunctive therapy.

In all cases a rapid reduction in dose rate or too sudden a change in treatment can result in relapse and recurrence of seizures.

Drug interactions are common between anticonvulsants and antibiotics, antacids, theophylline, cardiac drugs, steroids and antirheumatics. Phenothiazines (e.g. acepromazine), anthelminthics (e.g. piperazine and mebendazole) and metoclopramide administration may lower the seizure threshold and precipitate seizures in a stable case.

The incidence of seizures may be altered by the presence of concurrent disease – see Table 3.5. For this reason routine screening is advisable in geriatric patients with seizures.

Table 3.5 Concurrent diseases which may alter the incidence of seizures in older animals.

Gastroenteritis
Hepatic disease
Renal disease
Pneumonia
Metabolic disorders

METABOLIC ENCEPHALOPATHIES

Disorders of metabolism can induce disturbances in brain function which manifest as neurological deficits or excitation.

The brain consumes a large amount of energy (from glucose) and much of this is used to maintain the resting membrane potential of cells by the sodium-potassium pump. If available oxygen or glucose concentrations fall the pump fails and the membrane potential falls towards the threshold producing discharges and seizures. Further reductions in energy metabolism cause cell damage and loss and, if vital areas of the brain are involved, death may result.

Metabolic encephalopathies affect the brain diffusely but the cerebral cortex has the highest metabolic requirement so clinical signs are usually associated with cortical signs such as behavioural changes, changes in consciousness (depression or excitation), motor deficits and seizures. Thiamin deficiency (which is uncommon and can occur at any age) causes brainstem signs such as nystagmus.

Alterations in serum concentrations of calcium, sodium, potassium, magnesium or zinc can disturb normal neurological functions as can serum osmolarity and water balance. Cerebral oedema may occur if the serum is hypo-osmolar and also if a chronic hyperosmolar state is reversed too rapidly using intravenous fluids.

Endogenously produced toxins may alter brain metabolism and alter neurotransmission by affecting neurotransmitter synthesis or by producing 'false neurotransmitters'.

A full clinical work-up is needed to diagnose the underlying condition, including a detailed neurological examination. See Table 3.6 for a list of important causes that should be ruled out.

Table 3.6 Common causes of metabolic encephalopathy in ageing animals.

Liver failure – including cirrhosis
Renal failure – uraemia
Paraneoplastic disease – including lymphosarcoma
Secondary hyperparathyroidism – especially renal
Pyometra in bitches
Hypoglycaemia – e.g. insulinoma or insulin overdose
Hyperglycaemia – e.g. diabetes mellitus
Hypothyroidism
Heart failure – causing hypoxia
Respiratory disease – causing hypoxia
Dehydration – any cause
Addison's disease
Acid–base imbalance

1. Hepatic encephalopathy

Encephalopathy secondary to liver disease is seen most commonly in young animals with portocaval shunts, but it is also seen in old animals with advanced hepatic disease. In the presence of severely reduced liver function many toxins including ammonia, mercaptans, short chain fatty acids, indoles, skatoles and biologic amines accumulate in the circulation, brain and CSF. Ammonia is produced mainly by bacterial breakdown of protein and amino acids in the colon from where it is transported via the portal circulation and converted to urea by the liver. Mercaptans are produced by bacteria from methionine and short chain fatty acids are produced by bacterial action on dietary fat and they accumulate because they are not cleared by the liver. There is a shift in the ratio of circulating aromatic : aliphatic amino acids and these can act as false neurotransmitters in the CNS.

The neurological signs may be exacerbated by feeding a high protein diet. The other signs are those typically seen in liver disease.

Diagnosis is based upon clinical signs (Table 3.7) and evidence of liver disease or reduced liver function. Liver enzymes will only be elevated in the presence of active liver damage so liver function tests are preferred in older animals, particularly if cirrhosis is suspected. There are three main liver function tests, the bromosulphophthalein (BSP) clearance test, the ammonia tolerance test and bile acid estimation. The latter is now readily

Table 3.7 Clinical signs associated with hepatic encephalopathy.

Neurological signs
  Behavioural changes
  Aggression
  Depression
  Seizures
  Circling
  Head pressing
  Ataxia
  Blindness
  Coma
  Death

Other signs
  Weight loss
  Anorexia
  Diarrhoea
  Vomiting
  Pica
  Polydipsia
  Polyuria
  Ascites
  Jaundice

available, is reliable and the simplest test to perform and is recommended by the author.

It is usual to check plasma bile acid concentrations after fasting and 2 hours following feeding. Normal ranges are as follows (based upon enzymatic test):

Dogs   < 30 μmol/l after 12 hour fast
       < 50 μmol/l 2 hours after feeding

Cats   < 25 μmol/l after 12 hour fast
       < 30 μmol/l 2 hours after feeding.

Impaired liver function results in higher than normal bile acid concentrations.

Dietary management is the treatment of choice with a diet having the following characteristics:

(1) relatively low in protein content
(2) increased aromatic : aliphatic amino acid ratio
(3) moderate not a high fat content
(4) high essential to non-essential fatty acid ratio
(5) energy provided primarily in the form of carbohydrates as simple sugars
(6) high digestibility
(7) feed multiple small meals throughout the day.

Overfeeding should be avoided to minimise faecal residue and so reduce ammonia production due to bacterial degradation. Ammonia production can also be reduced by giving a lactulose enema – 30% lactulose to 70% water infused into the colon at 20–30 ml/kg body weight for 20–30 min. This is repeated until the pH of evacuated fluid is 6.0 or less.

Antibiotics effective against the urease-producing bacteria found in the colon (e.g. neomycin, metronidazole or ampicillin) may also reduce ammonia production.

2. *Hypoglycaemia*

The brain needs glucose as an energy source and hypoglycaemia may cause collapse, seizures, coma and death. In older animals hypoglycaemia may occur secondary to insulinomas, liver disease or sepsis/endotoxaemia.

Insulinomas

These are insulin-secreting tumours of the islet cells in the pancreas. They occur most frequently in dogs over 5 years of age, are usually malignant and spread locally. The hyperinsulinaemia that results causes episodic weakness or fainting due to hypoglycaemia. The signs are most severe in animals with concomitant impaired liver function.

Hyperinsulinaemia in the presence of hypoglycaemia is a useful indicator of the diagnosis because hypoglycaemia usually inhibits insulin production.

Surgical treatment may be successful in cases in which the insulinoma is localised to one area of the pancreas and when metastatic spread has not occurred.

Liver disease
The liver is responsible for gluconeogenesis and the maintenance of circulating blood glucose concentrations. If hepatic function is impaired hypoglycaemia may result.

Sepsis or endotoxaemia
Particularly as a consequence of pyometra, pyothorax, abscessation or a Gram-negative septicaemia.

3. *Hyperglycaemia*
Weakness and collapse may accompany hyperglycaemia which is usually caused by diabetes mellitus but which may also be associated with hyperadrenocorticism (particularly in the cat), hyperthyroidism (occurs in less than 10% of cats with this disorder), and obesity.

4. *Hyperkalaemia*
Hyperkalaemia may result from acidosis, hypoadrenocorticism, renal failure (oliguric) and massive tissue injury. Almost all clinical cases of hyperkalaemia result from a decreased ability to excrete potassium.

Affected animals present with neurological signs of muscle weakness and depressed reflexes. ECG abnormalities become apparent at circulating potassium concentrations above 7 mmol/l and death from cardiac arrest occurs when levels reach 10–12 mmol/l (Bush 1991).

5. *Hypokalaemic polyneuropathy*
Old cats are susceptible to develop potassium depletion due to urinary losses and the extracellular potassium depletion that results alters muscle cell membrane potential causing generalised muscle weakness. Hypokalaemia is defined as concentrations < 3.5 mmol potassium/l.

The presence of clinical signs associated with hypokalaemia (see Table 3.8) in an old cat should prompt a search for an underlying cause such as renal disease, gastrointestinal disorders, hyperaldosteronism or malnutrition.

Table 3.8 Clinical signs of hypokalaemia in cats.

Ventroflexion of the neck (similar to that which accompanies thiamin deficiency)
Poor exercise tolerance
Muscle pain
Excessive salivation
Crying

Treatment is 8–10 mmol potassium/day orally or 2–5 g (0.5–1 teaspoons) when given as potassium chloride (salt substitute) mixed in food. A complete balanced diet should be fed and clinical signs usually improve within 3 days. Potassium supplementation should not be given at the same time as special diets (e.g. Prescription Diet h/d – Hill's Pet Nutrition) which already contain an adequate amount of potassium.

6. Hypercalcaemia

Hypercalcaemia decreases cell membrane permeability in nervous tissue, reduces excitability and induces weakness and muscle wasting. The presence of hypercalcaemia in older animals should prompt a search for an underlying cause such as malignancy (particularly lymphosarcoma or anal gland adenocarcinoma), primary or secondary hyperparathyroidism, hypoadrenocorticism or renal failure. Severe acidosis may also be associated with an hypercalcaemia.

7. Hypocalcaemia

In the presence of inadequate extracellular calcium, neuromuscular cell membranes become unstable resulting in uncontrolled generalised muscular contractions (fasciculations) typical of hypocalcaemia tetany. Other neurological signs include weakness, trembling, ataxia and seizures. Exercise or excitement often exacerbate these signs. Other signs include polydipsia and polyuria.

Hypocalcaemia may be a complication of advanced renal failure and it also occurs in primary hypoparathyroidism, acute pancreatitis and severe protein-losing enteropathy.

When interpreting a laboratory result of hypocalcaemia (< 2.2 mmol/l) blood albumin concentrations should always be measured because hypoalbuminaemia will reduce total serum calcium and diagnostic laboratories usually measure and report total serum calcium although only the ionized calcium is physiologically active.

8. Hyponatraemia

Neurological signs of hyponatraemia include lethargy, depression, and nausea. Other signs include decreased cardiac output, hypovolaemia, hypotension and shock.

Hyponatraemia (< 140 mmol/l dog; < 145 mmol/l cat) occurs due to increased sodium loss, overhydration or increased water intake. Most commonly it occurs in hypoadrenocorticism (Addison's disease) due to hypoaldosteronism, in severe vomiting/diarrhoea, in end stage renal failure, diabetes mellitus, psychogenic polydipsia, and following diuretic therapy or overzealous fluid therapy.

Care is needed in interpreting laboratory results because hyperlipidaemia and hyperproteinaemia may both cause false low plasma sodium levels.

9. Hypercatecholaminaemia
Increased circulating concentrations of catecholamines cause neurological signs including weakness, trembling, seizures and head pressing. Other signs include hypotension or hypertension, epistaxis and retinal haemorrhages, tachycardia and tachydysrhythmias.

Increased secretion of adrenaline or nor-adrenaline occurs with tumours of the adrenal medulla (phaeochromocytoma) and can be intermittent or persistent.

10. Hyperadrenocorticism
Episodic weakness or collapse may be associated with the muscle weakness that occurs in hyperadrenocorticism (Cushing's disease). Sometimes affected animals develop myotonia with stiffness and muscle hypertrophy which forms a dimple when percussed. The myotonia can be confirmed by electromyogram.

11. Hypothyroidism
Hypothyroidism is sometimes associated with peripheral neuropathies and myopathy resulting in lethargy and poor exercise tolerance with episodic weakness and collapse. Obesity and/or muscle wasting may also be present.

12. Ischaemic neuropathy secondary to thromboembolism
Aortic embolism is a common sequel to cardiomyopathy in cats. Obstruction of arterial blood supply and release of vasoactive substances (e.g. 5-HT) locally prevents collateral supply from developing resulting in ischaemia and peripheral nerve axon degeneration and demyelination. Nerve regeneration can occur if circulation is re-established and neurological recovery usually takes place over a 2–3 week period.

Affected cats present with acute paresis or paralysis and sometimes with acute hindleg pain. Hindlimb reflexes may be suppressed or absent, femoral pulses are weak or absent and the distal limbs are cold to the touch.

Treatment is aimed at the primary problem and include analgesics in the first 24–48 hours, antiserotonin (5-HT) drugs (e.g. cyproheptadine) or low-dose acepromazine to improve circulation, and the use of aspirin (dose 25 mg every 3 days) to reduce platelet aggregation.

PERIPHERAL POLYNEUROPATHIES

Neuropathies can occur secondary to multisystemic disorders (e.g. neoplasia, diabetes mellitus) so a full clinical examination is necessary (see Table 3.9 for presenting signs). In older animals it may be difficult to differentiate poor proprioception from severe muscle weakness. (See Wheeler 1989 for a review of how to perform a thorough neurological examination.)

Table 3.9 Presenting signs in peripheral neuropathy.

Ataxia
Muscle atrophy
Hyporeflexia/hypotonia or paresis
Difficulty rising
The muscle weakness may be progressive, usually affects the hindlimbs before the forelimbs and is not exercise dependent
Loss of bark (neuropathy of the recurrent laryngeal nerve)
Megaoesophagus
Megacolon

NEOPLASIA

Central nervous system

Brain tumours can occur at any age but the incidence is very rare in animals under 5 years of age (Skerritt 1989). They are usually focal lesions and cause neurological signs directly related to the site at which they occur.

Localisation of brain tumours can be achieved from a complete neurological examination and the use of modern imaging techniques particularly computerised tomography (CT scans) and magnetic resonance imaging (MRI). Plain radiography is rarely helpful unless the tumour involves the bony parts of the cranium causing osteolysis or new bone deposition, and the use of contrast studies (positive or negative) alone is less reliable than CT or MRI. Many brain tumours produce 'hot spots' that can be detected by scintigraphy and photon emission computed tomography.

Meningiomas are the most common form of brain tumour in dogs and cats. In the dog these and gliomas are often locally invasive, and gliomas are particularly aggressive. Some brain tumours are accessible to surgery and, if benign and well described, may be successfully removed, e.g. meningiomas in cats, but the prognosis is guarded. Radiotherapy and chemotherapy have also been reported to lead to remission in some patients.

Spine

Spinal tumours can occur at any age but (with the exception of lymphomas) are most prevalent in older animals. They may cause pain or neurological signs which are usually insidious in onset. Spinal tumours are uncommon in dogs but account for up to 50% of cats with spinal disease, though many of these are lymphosarcoma in young individuals.

CSF examination is sometimes helpful, but myelography is usually needed to identify the site of the lesion.

Extradural tumours are usually primary bone neoplasms and occasionally secondary (e.g. from a prostatic carcinoma). In cats lymphosarcoma is the most common extradural tumour. Radiographic findings may include new bone deposition, bone loss or vertebral collapse. Surgery is possible for some tumours and medical treatment and/or radiotherapy for others.

Intradural neoplasms are usually either:

(1) meningiomas which in dogs occur most often in the cervical spine where they may be amenable to surgery; or
(2) nerve sheath tumours including neurofibromas and neurosarcomas which often occur in the brachial plexus and are difficult to remove surgically.

Primary intramedullary tumours are the least common. They are usually glial cell tumours or result from secondary metastatic spread.

The prognosis for patients with spinal tumours is guarded.

Peripheral nerves

Neoplasia of the brachial plexus are most prevalent in middle-aged and old animals and in dogs they are most often nerve sheath tumours, e.g. schwannomas, neuromas and neurofibromas. They are usually slow growing but are locally invasive and though they rarely spread to the lungs the prognosis is poor.

In dogs a mean age of 7.4 years has been reported for brachial plexus tumours (Sharp 1989). Most of the dogs were medium or large breeds and they all presented initially with unilateral intractable foreleg lameness or paresis with muscle atrophy and pain. The spinatus muscles over the scapular were most often involved. Over 45% had radiological or clinical evidence of spinal cord compression or invasion and often a small mass was palpable in the axilla. Horner's syndrome may occur in conjunction with these tumours in both dogs and cats.

Diagnosis

Biopsy of the tumour tissue which is hard and discoloured grey or off-white is possible during exploration of the plexus (Sharp 1989).

Treatment

In dogs with spinal cord involvement dorsal laminectomy is recommended to confirm the diagnosis and assess for surgical removal by a craniolateral approach (Sharp 1988). If the proximal border of the tumour can be identified high limb amputation with removal of local spinal nerves is the treatment of choice as local excision will usually result in severe neurological deficits and local recurrence of the tumour.

Prognosis

Guarded. Local recurrence is common.

RETICULOSIS

Reticulosis is an uncommonly diagnosed condition of adult dogs which causes neurological signs either suggestive of a focal lesion with unilateral signs, or with multifocal signs, including hyperaesthesia. These signs are usually slowly progressive. Severe visual deficits may also be associated with reticulosis.

CSF examination may help in diagnosis though the neurological signs are usually non-specific. On histological examination the disease is characterised by perivascular mononuclear cell infiltration with proliferation of histiocyte and microglial cellular elements.

Three forms of the disease have been defined cytologically:

(1) granulomatous reticulosis (or granulomatous meningoencephalitis)
(2) neoplastic reticulosis and
(3) microgliomatosis.

Prednisolone at 1–2 mg/day orally has been recommended as treatment for this condition but the long-term prognosis is poor.

SPINAL DISEASE

There are several diseases that may involve the spinal canal producing clinical signs including neurological deficits and these need to be differentiated. Radiography is important in reaching an accurate diagnosis and myelography is usually needed to identify space occupying lesions. Animals with gait abnormalities should also have non-neurological causes eliminated including osteoarthritis (or degenerative joint disease), hip dysplasia, bilateral osteochondritis dessicans and generalised bone disease, e.g. renal secondary hyperparathyroidism.

Discospondylitis

Discospondylitis may occur at any age and occurs most frequently in the cervical spine or at the lumbosacral junction. It is an inflammatory process (usually secondary to bacterial infection) of the intervertebral disc space which extends into the vertebral bodies either side and encroaches on the spinal canal. The diagnosis is confirmed by radiology and it needs to be differentiated from spondylosis which is a common incidental radiographic finding in older dogs.

Cervical spondylopathy usually occurs in an earlier age (up to 7 years in Dobermans).

Degenerative disc disease

Degenerative disc disease is common in young chondrodystrophic dogs and clinical signs associated with disc degeneration are unusual in geriatric patients of these breeds. In other large breed dogs the condition is more likely to be seen in middle-aged or older animals and they usually present with a gradually progressive hindleg ataxia and paresis. Anti-inflammatory drugs are the treatment of choice, and surgery is less likely to be successful in these patients than in young animals with acute disc prolapse. Sometimes there is a concurrent degenerative myelopathy.

Chronic degenerative radiculomyopathy

Most central and peripheral myopathies occur in young animals, but chronic degenerative radiculomyelopathy (CDRM) is frequently seen in elderly male German shepherd dogs and it is occasionally seen in other breeds. There is degeneration of the lumbar dorsal columns, fasciculus gracilis, lateral corticospinal tract and around the ventromedian fissure of the white matter of the cord. Lesions also involve the dorsal spinal roots and the thoracolumbar grey matter and nucleus gracilis show asytrocytic sclerosis. These degenerative changes are typical of a 'dying-back' disease (Griffiths and Duncan 1975).

The cause is unknown although vitamin B12 (cobalamin) deficiency has been suggested by some workers.

Diagnosis is based upon the presenting clinical signs (Table 3.10) and absence of a space occupying spinal lesion on myelography. Treatment is symptomatic, for example the provision of boots to protect the dorsa of the feet and there is no treatment that can reverse the neurological deficit.

Table 3.10 Clinical signs of CDRM.

Chronic progressive ataxia with paresis and loss of proprioception but no loss of pain sensation.
Excessive wearing of the dorsum of the claws (often with skin abrasions) is usually present due to the feet being dragged along the ground.
Flexing the hindpaw with its dorsum to the ground fails to elicit a normal placing reflex and turning the dog in a tight circle causes affected dogs to criss-cross their legs and trip themselves up.

Lumbosacral spondylopathy

There are a number of pathological changes that may occur at the lumbosacral junction leading to signs of low back pain or hyperaesthesia with decreased ability to exercise, difficulty in rising, and sometimes faecal or urinary incontinence. The signs are usually bilateral and weak hock flexion is the main neurological deficit (Denny *et al.* 1982). Large breed working dogs are most often affected though a similar condition has been reported in smaller toy breeds.

The aetiopathogenesis may be due to spinal stenosis, disc protrusion, spondylosis deformans or discospondylitis. Myelography, epidurography, transosseus venography or CT scan are useful for differentiating the cause and electrophysiological testing (EMG) is also helpful.

Decompressive surgical treatment (dorsal laminectomy or foramenotomy) is reported to provide good success, and antibiotic treatment is required for discospondylitis.

VESTIBULAR DISEASE

Both adult cats and dogs can present with acute onset severe vestibular signs including head tilt, circling, leaning and nystagmus In both species the condition is frequently misdiagnosed as 'stroke' although post-mortem examinations of the brain in such cases have failed to detect the presence of haemorrhages or infarcts.

The aetiopathogenesis of this syndrome is unknown but it needs to be differentiated from vestibular signs associated with infection (particularly from otitis externa/interna/media, or haemotogenous spread), toxicity (particularly antibiotics such as neomycin, streptomycin and gentamicin), nutritional deficiency (e.g. thiamin deficiency in cats) or neoplasia. Vestibular signs associated with neoplasia are usually slowly progressive and refractory to treatment.

No specific treatment can be recommended but in both species the condition is self-limiting. Dogs are usually normal within 1–2 weeks, cats in 2–3 weeks.

REFERENCES AND FURTHER READING

Arce, V., Lima, L., Tresguerres, N. & Devesa, J.A.F. (1990) Synergistic effect of growth hormone-releasing hormone (GHRH) and clonidine in stimulating GH release in young and old dogs. *Brain Research*, **537**, 359–62.

Bush, B.M. (1991) *Interpretation of Laboratory Results for Small Animal Clinicians.* Blackwell Scientific Publications, Oxford.

Cella, S.G. *et al.* (1987) Prolonged fasting or clonidine can restore the defective growth hormone secretion in old dogs. *Acta Endocrinologica (Copenhagen),* **121**, 177–84.

Cella, S.G. *et al.* (1992) Combined administration of GHRH and clonidine restores the defective GH secretion in old dogs. *Neuroendocrinology* (in press).

Cummings, B.J., Honsberger, P.E., Afagh, A.J., *et al.* (1993) Cognitive function and Alzheimer's-like pathology in the aged canine. II. *Neuropathol Neurobiol Aging*, **14**, 547.

Cocola, F. *et al.* (1976) A rapid radioimmunassay method for growth hormone in dog plasma. *Proceedings of the Society for Experimental Biology and Medicine*, **151**, 140–5.

D'Costa, A.P., Ingram, R.L., Lenham, J.E. & Sonntag, W.E. (1993) The regulation and mechanisms of action of growth hormone and insulin-like growth factor 1 during normal ageing. *Journal of Reproduction and Fertility Supplement*, **46**, 87–98.

Denny, H.R., Gibbs, C. & Holt, P.E. (1982) The diagnosis and treatment of cauda equina lesions in the dog. *Journal of Small Animal Practice*, **23**, 425.

Greene, C.E. & Appel, M.J. (1990) Canine distemper. In: *Infectious Diseases of the Dog and Cat* (ed. C.E. Greene), pp. 226–41. W.B. Saunders, Philadelphia.

Griffiths, I.R. & Duncan, I.D. (1975) Chronic degenerative radiculomyopathy in the dog. *Journal of Small Animal Practice*, **16**, 461–71.

Meites, J. (1993) Anti-ageing interventions and their neuroendocrine aspects in mammals. *Journal of Reproduction and Fertility Supplement*, **46**, 1–9.

Morys *et al.* (1994) *NeuroReport*, **5**, 1825.

Schwartz-Porsche, D. (1992) Management of refractory seizures. In: *Kirk's Current Veterinary Therapy XI: Small Animal Practice* (eds R.W. Kirk & J.D. Bonogura), pp. 986–91. W.B. Saunders, Philadelphia.

Sharp, N.J.H. (1988) Craniolateral approach to the canine brachial plexus. *Veterinary Surgery*, **17**, 18.

Sharp, N.J.H.(1989) Neurological deficits in one limb. In: *Manual of Small Animal Neurology* (ed. S.J. Wheeler), p. 183. BSAVA Publications, Cheltenham.

Skerritt, G.C. (1989) Brain disorders in dogs and cats. In: *Manual of Small Animal Neurology* (ed. S.J. Wheeler). BSAVA Publications, Cheltenham.

Wheeler, S.J. (1989) *Manual of Small Animal Neurology.* British Small Animal Veterinary Association, Cheltenham.

Chapter 4
THE SPECIAL SENSES

KEY POINTS

(1) Ageing changes may occur in all sensory organs leading to a gradual reduction in sensitivity and response to external stimuli.
(2) If the loss of sensory perception occurs gradually owners may not notice that the sense is being lost in their pet.
(3) Ageing changes are irreversible so any age-related loss of sensory perception is permanent. Adjusting the lifestyle of the pet can minimise the effects of loss of the special senses.

4.1 AGEING CHANGES IN MAJOR SENSE ORGANS

NOSE

Loss of smell may occur with advancing age but there is no evidence that this is a significant problem in old cats and dogs. In part this may be because recognition of loss of smell is a problem for owners and veterinary clinicians because there is no change in behaviour pattern apart from reduced appetite which specifically indicates that such a loss is present.

Age-related diseases

There are a number of age-related diseases that may affect the nose, the most important of which are intranasal neoplasia and chronic rhinitis.

Neoplasia

The average age of dogs and cats with intranasal neoplasia is reported to be 9 years. The condition is less common in cats. In the dog most neoplasms are adenocarcinomas. In cats benign polyps which extend to the nasopharynx are also seen.

Nasal tumours are locally invasive and cause destruction of bone which can be identified on radiography and loss of the fine trabecular pattern of the nasal turbinates is a sign of early nasal neoplasia. This is best demonstrated on intra-oral dorsoventral projections. Spread to local tissues including the eye and brain is common. Clinical signs include sneezing, nasal discharges including epistaxis, obstructed air flow when breathing and later deformity of the face or clinical signs associated with spread to adjacent structures such as the brain.

Diagnosis is based on clinical signs, radiography and excisional biopsy. Flushing the nasal cavity to extract exfoliated cells for cytological examination might also be a useful technique in some cases.

Treatments that have been reported to be successful in some cases include surgery, surgery with radiotherapy and radiotherapy alone but the prognosis is always poor–guarded.

Chronic rhinitis

Chronic rhinitis may be a consequence of bacterial, viral or fungal infection, trauma or foreign bodies. Only about 50% of cases will respond to treatment and the prognosis is poor–guarded. Treatment is dependent upon an accurate diagnosis of the underlying cause. Even if microbiological culture and sensitivity indicates a specific therapeutic approach complete success may not be achieved because the infection is in a cavity, and for this reason some clinicians prefer to flush through trephined holes or a nasal bone flap – particularly for the treatment of aspergillus or infections extending into sinuses. Partial or complete turbinectomy can be performed in some cases, and some authors advocate complete bilateral extirpation of all turbinate tissues (Gourley and Vasseur 1985).

EAR

Apparent loss of hearing is commonly seen in old dogs, but rarely reported in old cats. Owners notice that their pet is slow to respond to auditory stimuli such as the noise of them being called, whistles, the sound of the owner entering the room, or loud bangs such as doors slamming or fireworks. Sometimes owners can recognise complete deafness when their dog fails to respond to all auditory stimulation but does respond immediately to visual recognition.

Chronic inflammation can lead to thickening and pigmentation of the skin lining the ear canal and this may lead to narrowing of the external auditory meatus. This in itself may not cause a significant impairment in hearing.

EYE

There are many age-related changes which can be recognised in eyes including the following:

Eyelid papillomas

Papillomas or warts are very common in old dogs – particularly on the eyelid margins. Excision is indicated when they impinge on the cornea causing irritation, inflammation or self-trauma. Melanomas and carcinomas occur occasionally, but they are rare.

Cysts of the gland of Moll

These cysts are usually small and have a vesicular appearance. They do not cause clinical problems but can be surgically excised if necessary.

Increased tear viscosity

Increasing tear viscosity will reduce the rate of flow of tears across the corneal surface, thus reducing the ability of the tear film to wash away particulate matter that might collect on the surface.

Decreased lysozyme activity

Reduced lysozyme activity may lead to increased susceptibility to infection.

Corneal pigmentation

Corneal pigmentation with melanin is a common condition in dogs and is usually secondary to inflammation or some other corneal or uveal disease. If heavy pigmentation is present it will result in impaired vision.

If a primary cause cannot be identified (e.g. entropion, trauma, distichiasis, trichiasis, neoplasia (melanoma), keratitis sicca etc.) senile corneal degeneration should be considered as a possible cause.

Treatment depends upon the underlying cause. If surgical correction of a primary cause is not possible, corticosteroid therapy can be successfully employed in most cases. Superficially pigmented areas can be excised surgically.

Corneal lipid deposits

Corneal dystrophies are seen in older animals and usually present as bilateral, progressive, degenerative lesions. Lipid deposits may appear in the corneal stroma, and sometimes other materials can become deposited, e.g. calcium. Treatment is rarely indicated but an underlying cause should be sought (e.g. hyperlipidaemia, hypercalcaemia) and treated if possible.

Iris atrophy

This is rare but can lead to blockage of the drainage angle resulting in glaucoma.

Nuclear sclerosis

With advancing age fibres near the centre of the lens become compressed and this, with concomitant loss of water causes an increase in density of the lens nucleus (called sclerosis) which gives a blue-grey tinge to the lens. Nuclear sclerosis affects most dogs over 6 years of age to some degree or other, but transmission of light to the retina is not affected, the fundus is visible on ophthalmoscopic examination because the discoloured lens is still translucent and vision is not seriously impaired. No treatment is needed although there have been unsubstantiated anecdotal reports of nuclear sclerotic lesions disappearing following a change in diet from an adult maintenance ration to one formulated specifically for old dogs.

Cataracts

Senile cataracts are common in dogs and most dogs over 9 years will have some evidence of cataract formation. Usually the opacity progresses slowly and it may affect the nuclear or cortical part of the lens. They are usually blue-grey initially progressing to yellow or even brown with maturity. Despite the obvious opacity vision is often not severely impaired.

(1) Nuclear cataracts form as a result of the normal process of nuclear sclerosis.
(2) Cortical cataracts are most commonly seen in old dogs and are due to the accumulation of fluid within the lens cortex.
(3) Diabetic cataracts may appear earlier in life (from 2 years of age). They are usually bilateral and progress rapidly. The lens changes may be reversed if treated early enough.
(4) Punctate cataracts have been reported in association with hypo-calcaemia, hypoparathyroidism and renal insufficiency.

Impaired vision due to cataract formation is manifest as bizarre behavioural changes including barking at imaginary objects.

There is no satisfactory medical treatment for cataracts and various surgical approaches (e.g. extraction, phaecoemulsification) have been recommended.

Asteroid hyalosis

Calcium deposits called asteroid bodies are sometimes seen in the vitreous of ageing animals. They are usually only present in one eye and appear like small white round deposits. The cause is unknown, they do not cause problems and do not require treatment.

Vitreous liquefaction

This degenerative change is often seen in old animals and those that have cataracts.

Loss of rods and cones

An age-related decrease in numbers of rods and cones results in decreased visual acuity, and could result ultimately in visual impairment.

Retinal detachment

Retinal detachment is common in cats and an occasional finding in dogs. It is often bilateral and is usually secondary to hypertension such as occurs in chronic renal failure. Detachment can be slow or sudden and total detachment results in blindness.

Cystoid retinal degeneration

Cystoid retinal degeneration is common, particularly in the region of the ora serata, and it is regarded as a normal ageing process.

Neoplasia

Retinal neoplasia is rare and usually secondary to uveal tract neoplasia when it does occur. Uveal tract tumours are more common and most involve the ciliary body or extensive areas of the uveal tract. Most are malignant and pigmented neoplasms are usually melanomas. Usually only one eye is affected. Differentiating pigment changes of the iris from malignant melanoma can be difficult or even impossible. Because of this, and because melanoma within the eye tend to metastasise slowly (unlike malignant melanoma of oral origin), enucleation should only be performed when the pigmented mass grows rapidly, it develops an irregular contour, causes local discomfort or there are intraocular haemorrhages. When metastasis does occur it can be to the brain, lungs or elsewhere in the body.

In cats lymphosarcoma of the iris may be associated with positive feline leukaemia virus (FeLV) status.

The net effect of slowly progressive age-related changes leads initially to loss of visual acuity then to visual impairment and finally to blindness. Full ophthalmological examination is needed and should be incorporated into any geriatric screening programme. It should include ophthalmoscopy, assessment of pupillary reflexes and the menace reflex.

TONGUE

Loss of taste sensation may occur with advancing age but there is no evidence that this is a common problem in cats and dogs. The likely effects of such a loss would be reduced appetite and some authors have described malnutrition in surgical cases involving the nasal passages.

Neoplasia

Neoplasia of the tongue is uncommon in dogs, but there is a relatively high incidence in cats. In the cat most neoplasms are squamous cell carcinoma, and others include fibrosarcoma, papilloma and haemangioma. In dogs malignant melanoma is the most serious as it is highly malignant, the fibrosarcoma and squamous cell carcinoma are also seen. All carry a poor prognosis. If localised surgical excision may be possible (e.g. papillomas) and in cats radiotherapy has been suggested as the best treatment for squamous cell carcinoma. Some haemangiomas are corticosteroid responsive, but there is no satisfactory treatment for fibrosarcoma though radiotherapy or hyperthermia may be helpful in some cases.

Uraemia

Ulceration around the lingual margin and severe halitosis is associated with advanced uraemia due to renal failure.

4.2 SUMMARY

With advancing age most cats and dogs probably lose some of their sense of smell, hearing, sight and taste, however they cope very well in familiar surroundings and owners are unlikely to recognise serious behavioural or other problems unless there is a total loss of sense, e.g. blindness, deafness.

REFERENCES AND FURTHER READING

Gourley, I.M. & Vasseur, P.B. (eds) (1985) Nasal cavity, paranasal sinuses, larynx and ears. In: *General Small Animal Surgery*. J.B. Lippincott, Philadelphia.

Chapter 5
URINARY TRACT

KEY POINTS

(1) Chronic renal failure is common in old cats and dogs and is a major cause of death.

(2) It is generally accepted that chronic renal failure is a slowly progressive condition whatever the initial cause of the disease and it is believed that proper clinical management may delay or stop progression.

(3) Urinary incontinence and/or inappropriate urination is commonly reported in dogs and cats with advancing age, and is a major reason for euthanasia being requested by owners.

(4) Dietary management is an important management tool in urinary tract disorders.

(5) Screening for evidence of renal impairment is important before the administration of therapeutic agents or a general anaesthetic to old patients.

5.1 UPPER URINARY TRACT: AGE-RELATED CHANGES

The following changes have been reported to occur with advancing age (after Mosier 1988 and Breitschwerdt 1988):

- reduced renal size
- reduced number of nephrons
- reduced glomerular filtration rate (GFR)
- reduced renal plasma flow

- reduced tubular excretion
- reduced tubular reabsorption.

Compensated renal failure is present in many older animals. In one recent survey of 13 apparently healthy cats aged over 7 years of age *all* of them were found to have blood creatinine with/or without increased urea concentrations above the published normal range (Barber, P. 1995 personal communication), and in another survey of 1600 dogs aged over 5 years 22.4% were found to have evidence of azotaemia (Leibetseder & Neufeld, 1991). Recent studies at the Royal Veterinary College, University of London have been unable to detect an age-related decrease in GFR using non-invasive radioactive technetium.

Early detection of the presence of renal failure is desirable to facilitate early intervention in an attempt to delay or stop progression and also to identify individuals in which renal excretion of drugs may be impaired, and those at risk of developing acute renal failure if stressed by the administration of some drugs, e.g. non-steroidal anti-inflammatory drugs (NSAIDs), some antibiotics or the administration of a general anaesthetic.

5.2   DIETARY MANAGEMENT

Dietary management is very important in the management of renal disease in older animals due to the effect that diet has on:

- calorie intake
- renal blood flow
- uraemia
- nephrocalcinosis
- urine pH.

When considering the most appropriate dietary regimen for an individual case it is important to perform a full and detailed clinical examination, because renal disease may be associated with concomitant disease in other organ systems, e.g. pyometra (Stone *et al.* 1988) and heart failure (Ralston & Fox 1988) which may influence dietary choice.

Renal disease increases in incidence with increasing age (Muller-Peddinghaus & Trautwein 1977) and so it frequently occurs in individuals that also have compromised cardiac, hepatic or other organ function. The most serious disorder will usually be managed first.

Complications may even occur within the urinary tract itself. For example, renal failure precipitated by urinary tract obstruction due to a struvite urolith, presents the clinician with a dilemma, because the diet of choice for renal failure is not ideal for the management of struvite urolithiasis. In such circumstances the clinician needs to use his/her clinical judgement to manage the case most effectively.

Calorie intake

All animals have a requirement for energy which has to be met by dietary intake. The energy requirements of animals during their life cycle stages have been reasonably well established (NRC 1985; NRC 1986; Lewis *et al.* 1987) but the energy requirements of animals with renal disease have yet to be accurately determined.

Assessing the body weight of an animal is important in estimating the calorie requirements of an individual. A reduction in calorie intake should be considered for animals that are obese, and calorie intake should be increased for animals that are underweight. Cats and dogs with renal disease frequently present in a catabolic state and they need a high calorie intake to maintain body functions and to restore normal body weight. This may not be easy to achieve, as animals in a debilitated state or with azotaemia are frequently anorectic.

Uraemic animals may vomit any food that is eaten, and in the presence of concomitant gastrointestinal or hepatic dysfunction, ingestion may not guarantee adequate utilisation of the food. The diet for such cases should therefore be high in energy density and digestibility to minimise the amount of food that the animal has to digest and absorb. Feeding small volumes of food frequently (3–4 times daily) may improve utilisation.

Hand feeding, warming the food and sometimes the administration of diazepine drugs (e.g. diazepam at a dose rate of 2–14 mg/kg orally (dogs) *or* 1–2 mg/cat orally or 0.1–0.5 mg/cat given intravenously; or oxazepam at a dose rate of 2 mg/cat orally) may encourage eating in anorectic patients (Lewis *et al.* 1987). Diets claiming good palatability should be selected carefully to avoid those containing high levels of nutrients (e.g. salt) that might be contraindicated in the presence of renal disease.

Studies in man have demonstrated an improvement in ability to maintain nitrogen equilibrium by increasing the calorie intake of uraemic patients on a low-protein, high biological value protein diet (Hyne *et al.* 1972).

A high calorie-dense diet reduces the amount of food that has to be eaten to meet daily energy needs, and this can be helpful in reducing the total intake of specific nutrients that have to be controlled, e.g. phosphorus intake will be less if less food is eaten.

Cats, being obligate carnivores, have a high requirement for energy from dietary protein. In the presence of inadequate protein–calories a cat will breakdown its own body protein to produce energy, hence severe dietary protein restriction is not as feasible in the cat as it is in the dog.

Renal blood flow

Loss of renal function is commonly slow and progressive with a progressive fall in glomerular filtration rate (GFR) caused by increasing loss of functional nephrons. One mechanism by which this progress is believed to occur is the 'hyperfiltration theory' (Brenner *et al.* 1982). This theory is based upon the increased workload on functioning nephrons, in kidneys in which renal reserve has been lost due to injury. Under such circumstances surviving nephrons are subjected to intraglomerular hypertension and hyperperfusion which can result in glomerular injury (sclerosis) and further loss of function.

Ingestion of a meal causes a postprandial increase in renal perfusion and filtration and by cumulative effect this is thought to be responsible for hyperfiltration and the renal hypertrophy seen in animals maintained on high protein diets. In the dog changing from a carbohydrate to a meat diet increases renal blood flow and filtration rates by as much as 100% (Shannon *et al.* 1932; Pitts 1944). This increase in renal blood flow is thought to be mediated by a hormone (e.g. glucagon) or other factor (Rocha *et al.* 1972; Aoki *et al.* 1976; Johannesen *et al.* 1977).

In the presence of decreasing renal function, therefore, feeding a low protein diet is indicated to decrease further glomerular damage caused by the above effects on renal haemodynamics.

It has also been suggested that augmented intrarenal pressures and flows associated with ad libitum feeding might contribute to age-related glomerular sclerosis (Brenner *et al.* 1982), but whether or not diet induced changes can result ultimately in disease, remains controversial.

In experimental models reducing dietary protein intake has been associated with decreased progression of renal haemodynamics (Hostetter *et al.* 1981) and improved longevity (Kleinknecht *et al.* 1979; Salusky *et al.* 1981). Other studies have demonstrated accelerated glomerulosclerosis in uninephrectomised rats fed high protein diets (Blatherwick & Medlar 1937; Lalich *et al.* 1975) and retardation of the progression of renal failure in rats (Farr & Smadel 1939; Neugarten *et al.* 1982; Friend *et al.* 1978), and in mice (Farr & Smadel 1939), by feeding a protein restricted diet.

Increasing glomerular pathology as evaluated by light microscopy (including glomerulosclerosis) has been reported in nephrectomised dogs fed increasing levels of dietary protein (Bovee *et al.* 1979; Robertson *et al.* 1986). Several studies in dogs with renal failure have shown that dietary protein restriction reduces proteinuria, an indicator of glomerular injury (Polzin *et al.* 1983; Polzin *et al.* 1984; Polzin & Osborne 1988) and recent studies show that glomerular hyperfiltration may promote the development of glomerular sclerosis in dogs with chronic renal failure (Polzin *et al.* 1988).

In humans a prospective, randomised study has recently been reported (Ihle *et al.* 1989) after which the authors concluded that dietary protein restrictions was effective in slowing the rate of progression of chronic renal failure.

Protein malnutrition has been shown to be unlikely to occur on a protein intake of more than 1.9 g protein/kg body weight per day in dogs with chronic renal failure (Polzin *et al.* 1991). Protein intake below this amount did not further reduce hyperfiltration and hence would be of no additional benefit in reducing glomerular injury.

Systemic hypertension has been reported in dogs with acute and sub-acute interstitial nephritis (Anderson & Fisher 1968) and in 58–93% of dogs with renal failure (Cowgill 1982; Weiser *et al.* 1971). The presence of systemic hypertension may result in intraglomerular hypertension, although it is not necessarily present for the development of the latter. Animals with renal insufficiency are unable to regulate sodium excretion properly, however net loss of sodium (sodium dumping) was not demonstrated in one study in which sodium intake was decreased abruptly in nephrectomised dogs (Schmidt *et al.* 1974). Currently it is recommended that the sodium intake for dogs and cats with renal disease be limited to 0.1–0.3% in dry matter, which is considerably less than the levels in most commercial pet foods (Lewis *et al.* 1987).

Sodium supplementation is contraindicated, though this was once commonly recommended.

Maintaining blood haemodynamics to avoid hypoperfusion and ischaemia is an important objective in the management and prevention of acute renal failure, and interestingly it has recently been suggested that limiting protein intake might reduce the susceptibility of renal tubular cells to nephrotoxic or ischaemic stress, such as occurs in renal failure (Andrews & Bates 1986; Polzin & Osborne 1990).

Uraemia is a common occurrence in renal disease, and urea itself may increase renal blood flow, thus having an effect on renal haemodynamics.

Uraemia

The uraemic syndrome results from an inability of the kidney to excrete nitrogenous waste products including urea, and other toxins. Reduction of dietary intake of protein reduces the quantity of circulating proteinaceous waste products and has been shown in many studies in rats, people and dogs to result in marked clinical improvement, increased survival and preserved renal function. A comprehensive reference list has been published (Lewis *et al.* 1987).

It has been shown that people (Walser & Mitch 1977) and dogs (Osborne 1980) with renal failure have a higher requirement for protein than normal individuals and the amount of protein needed will depend upon the severity of the renal dysfunction and the digestibility and quality of the protein in the food. The aim therefore is to feed sufficient high biologic value protein to meet the animal's requirements, but to maintain a blood urea level of 60 mg/dl (10 mmol/l) or less. Approximations of the amount of protein needed in dogs with renal failure to achieve this have been published (see Table 5.1).

Clinical signs attributable to uraemia should be controlled at a BUN of less than 60 mg/dl (10 mmol/l).

Table 5.1 Amount of dietary protein that will result in a BUN of 60 mg/dl (10 mmol/l) in a dog with renal failure.

Plasma creatinine (μmol/l)	Dietary protein intake (% dry matter)
310	25
354	19
397	14
442	10
486	7

(After Lewis *et al.* 1987)

Nephrocalcinosis

With decreasing renal function the kidney becomes less able to:

- degrade parathyroid hormone
- excrete phosphorus
- convert vitamin D to its active form.

Reduction in these activities results in bone demineralisation or osteodystrophy and mineral deposition in soft tissues, including the kidneys themselves, which further reduces function. This mineral deposition can occur at normal plasma calcium and phosphorus concentrations in damaged renal tissue, and it can be an early morphological abnormality in animals with renal insufficiency.

Dietary phosphorus restriction has been reported to reduce nephrocalcinosis and osteodystrophy even in mild renal insufficiency before increased plasma phosphorus levels (Maschio *et al.* 1980). Plasma phosphorus concentrations should be kept at 5.0 mg/dl (1.6 mmol/l) or less, and plasma calcium levels at 10 mg/dl (2.5 mmol/l) or more, with a solubility factor for the two of less than 55 (Massry 1980).

Phosphorus restriction significantly reduced the degree of tissue mineralisation in nephrectomised cats when compared with cats fed a normal diet (Ross *et al.* 1982), and high phosphorus intake in nephrectomised dogs resulted in hyperparathyroidism and severe bone demineralisation as compared with dogs with reduced phosphorus intake (Rutherford *et al.* 1977).

Studies in cats and dogs have demonstrated that phosphate binders are ineffective at the commonly used dosages if diets with unrestricted phosphorus content are fed.

Urine pH

Acidosis may occur with oliguria or severe polyuric renal failure and is due to reduced excretion of sulphates, phosphorus, organic acids, hydrogen and ammonium ions. Metabolic acidosis enhances osteodystrophy and protein catabolism.

Acidifying diets should be avoided in animals with renal failure.

Summary of dietary management

1. Chronic renal failure

Feed a diet that is:

- high in energy-density
- low in protein content (contains high biological value protein)
- low in phosphorus content
- low in sodium content
- buffered against acidosis.

e.g. Prescription Diet Canine or Feline k/d; Prescription Diet Canine u/d (Hill's Pet Nutrition).

2. Glomerular Disease (nephrotic syndrome)

Protein loss into the urine accompanies glomerular disease and may lead to hypoproteinaemia. Feed a diet with the same profile as that listed above for chronic renal failure. It used to be advised that extra high biological value protein in the form of whole egg or cottage cheese should be added if the animal developed hypoproteinaemia, however recent evidence suggests that increasing dietary intake of protein only results in increased urinary excretion. Furthermore the effect of the increased protein on renal haemodynamics (see above) might make this practice more harmful than beneficial.

5.3 LOWER URINARY TRACT: DISORDERS OF URINATION

Inappropriate urination is commonly reported to occur in older dogs and cats that have previously been house trained, and this behaviour change is frequently a reason for owners seeking euthanasia (Ruehl W.W., personal communication).

In some individuals the micturating reflex may be abnormal due to impaired neuromuscular function (either locally or in the CNS) with loss of conscious voluntary control of urination (Oliver 1987). In other cases the individual may be exhibiting behavioural changes due to senile changes in the CNS (see Chapter 3).

Urinary incontinence is common in old bitches and has been linked to ovarohysterectomy by some authors but the evidence from long-term studies have still to confirm such an association. Failure of the urethral sphincter mechanism is the underlying problem and some cases respond to oestrogen therapy (stilboestrol – orally at 0.1–1 mg daily for 3–5 days followed by weekly treatment has been recommended). Urethral tone can be improved by administering α-adrenergic stimulants (with or without concurrent use of oestrogens) and phenylpropanolamine is currently recommended at 1.5 mg/kg b.i.d. or 1 mg/kg t.i.d.

Involuntary voiding of urine may be primary (associated with a neuro-muscular disorder of the bladder) or secondary to a primary condition such as urinary tract infection or neoplasia. Although rare, primary detrusor muscle disorders may respond to anticholinergic drugs, e.g. propantheline at a dose rate of 7.5–15 mg t.i.d.

Any condition that causes bladder wall irritability (e.g. cystitis) can lead to frequent micturition which can easily be confused with incontinence by owners.

Urinary incontinence can be a sequel to urine retention for example due to urolithiasis, or spinal injury or disease.

Urethral disease

Urethral disorders are not common in old cats or dogs. Clinical signs are usually dysuria and haematuria. Obstruction may be caused by uroliths, foreign bodies or neoplasms. In male cats with feline urologic syndrome (FUS or feline lower urinary tract disease) urethral scarring and stenosis may be a complication following repeated attempts at catheterisation. If obstruction is prolonged urinary incontinence may be a complication once the obstruction is removed.

5.4   LOWER URINARY TRACT: PROSTATIC DISEASE

Diseases of the prostate are rare in cats but are common in older dogs and all may present with similar histories and clinical signs:

- pain – caudal abdomen on palpation or movement and on defaecation
- constipation
- straining – on defaecation or urination
- dysuria – common in humans but not very common in dogs.

Secondary complications include prostatitis (common in older dogs and one possible cause of intractable haematuria) and perineal rupture. It is important to differentiate benign hyperplasia (which is common) from prostate neoplasia (carcinoma) which is less common and life-threatening. Paraprostatic cysts are also seen occasionally and these may complicate the diagnosis. Radiography, ultrasound and physical examination are all useful diagnostic aids which can be further reinforced by prostatic washes or biopsy.

If prostatic carcinoma is suspected, survey radiographs should be performed to identify evidence of metastatic spread, especially to the lungs, and also to bone and lymph nodes. Surgical removal can be difficult but is successful in providing remission in some cases. Usually it is combined with castration. I have had some success with surgical excision and cryo-surgery on tissue that is difficult to resect locally.

For prostatic hyperplasia, castration with or without therapeutic agents such as stilboestrol is indicated. In old dogs that are an anaesthetic risk, medical treatment alone may be necessary.

Paraprostatic cysts (often there are more than one lying alongside the urinary bladder) are difficult to manage, there being no medical therapy, and surgical techniques such as excision and marsupialisation to provide permanent drainage being reported to have mixed success. I prefer to attempt surgical resection.

Prostatitis can be difficult to treat and quite often antibiotic therapy has to be continued for 6–8 weeks. Ideally the antibiotic of choice will be based upon culture and sensitivity tests and it is important that the diagnostic laboratory test for sensitivity is based upon urine concentrations of the drug and not just the blood concentrations achieved. A history of chronic haematuria or urinary tract infection in male dogs should always suggest the possibility of prostatitis.

There are three main differential diagnoses of prostatic disorders in old dogs (see Table 5.2).

Other, less common, prostatic disorders include prostatic cysts and trauma. Aids to diagnosis include:

Table 5.2 Main prostatic disorders in old dogs.

	Hypertrophy	Neoplasia	Prostatitis
Average age	90% over 5 years	90% over 8 years	Chronic form common in older dogs
Rectal palpation	Bilateral enlargement Often very large Usually smooth surfaced Often painful – but not in uncomplicated cases	Usually unilateral but may be bilateral Not usually as large as hypertrophy Usually firm and nodular	Painful
Treatment	Oestrogen therapy – temporary regression Castration	Prostatectomy – difficult but can be very successful (morbidity 30%, mortality 10%) ?Castration	Antibiosis based on culture and sensitivity (erythromycin, trimethoprim, lincomycin and chloramphenicol achieve good tissue penetration) ?Surgical drainage and flushing
Other comments	If oestrogen therapy does not induce regression – biopsy An age-related hormonal imbalance has been suggested as a cause*	Must radiograph and/ or use ultrasound to establish whether or not there is local metastasis (e.g. to the pelvis) or widespread metastasis (e.g. to lungs or liver)	Attempts at surgical drainage can lead to peritonitis Prostatic hypertrophy may predispose old dogs to develop prostatitis

* Dihydrotestosterone accumulates in hypertrophic canine (and human) prostates and dihydrotesterone and testosterone do not induce hypertrophy whereas 3 α-androstanediol and 17β-estradiol (both secreted by the testis) do produce hypertrophy. Furthermore antioestrogen drugs (e.g. tamoxifen) or antiandrogens (e.g. cyproterone) cause glandular atrophy in both spontaneous and experimental canine prostatic hypertrophy.

- radiography
- ultrasound
- biopsy
- prostatic massage/flushing.

REFERENCES AND FURTHER READING

Anderson, L.J. & Fisher, E.W. (1968) The blood pressure in canine interstitial nephritis. *Research in Veterinary Science*, **9**, 304–13.

Andrews, P.M. & Bates, S.B. (1986) Dietary protein prior to renal ischaemia dramatically affects postischaemic kidney function. *Kidney International*, **30**, 299–303.

Aoki, T.T., Brennan, M.F., Muller, W.A. *et al.* (1976) Amino acid levels across normal forearm muscle and splanchnic bed after a protein meal. *American Journal of Clinical Nutrition*, **29**, 340–50.

Blatherwick, N.R. & Medlar, E.M. (1937) Chronic nephritis in rats fed high protein diets. *Archives of Internal Medicine*, **59**, 572–96.

Bovee, K.C., Kronfeld, D.S., Ramberg, C. *et al.* (1979) Long-term measurement of renal function in partially nephrectomized dogs fed 56, 27 or 19% protein. *Investigative Urology*, **16**, 378.

Breitschwerdt, E.B. (1988) *Proceedings of Symposium on Clinical Conditions in the Older Cat and Dog*, The Royal Garden Hotel, London, 15 June 1988, p.15. Published by Hill's Pet Products Ltd, London.

Brenner, B.M., Meyer, T.W. & Hostetter, T.H. (1982) The role of hemodynamically mediated glomerular injury in the pathogenesis of progressive glomerular sclerosis in aging, renal ablation and intrinsic renal disease. *New England Journal of Medicine*, **307**, 652–59.

Cowgill, L.D. (1982) Renal insufficiency and diseases of the glomerulus. *Proceedings of the California Veterinary Medical Association* 94th Annual Seminar Oct 14–17.

Cowgill, L.D. (1983) Diseases of the kidney. In: *Textbook of Internal Medicine* (ed. S. Ettinger) 2nd edn, pp. 1793–1879.

Cowgill, L.D. & Spangler, W.L. (1981) Renal insufficiency in geriatric dogs. In: *Veterinary Clinics of North America Small Animal Practice*, **11**(4), 727–47.

European Society of Veterinary Nephrology and Urology (1988) *Proceedings of the 3rd Annual Symposium on Urolithiasis*. Barcelona, Spain.

Farr, L.E. & Smadel, J.D. (1939) The effect of dietary protein on the course of nephrotoxic nephritis in rats. *Journal of Experimental Medicine*, **70**, 615–27.

Friend, P.S., Fernandes, G. & Good, R.A. *et al.* (1978) Dietary restrictions early and late: effects on the nephropathy of the NZB × NZW mouse. *Laboratory Investigation*, **298**, 122–6.

Gaskell, C.J. (1979) *Studies on the feline urological syndrome*. PhD thesis, University of Bristol.

Hostetter, T.H., Olson, J.L., Rennke, H.G. *et al.* (1981) Hyperfiltration in remnant nephrons a potentially adverse response to renal ablation. *American Journal of Physiology*, **241**, F85–93.

Hyne, B.E.B., Fowell, E. & Lee, H.A. (1972) The effect of calorie intake on nitrogen balance in chronic renal failure. *Clinical Science*, **43**, 679–88.

Ihle, B.U. *et al.* (1989) The effect of protein restriction on the progression of renal insufficiency. *New England Journal of Medicine*, **321**, 1773–7.

Johannesen, J., Lie, M. & Kiil, F. (1977) Effect of glycine and glucagon on glomerular filtration and renal metabolic rates. *American Journal of Physiology*, **233**, F61–6.

Kleinknecht, C., Salusky, I., Broyer, M. & Gubler, M-C. (1979) Effect of various protein diets on growth, renal function and survival time of uraemic rats. *Kidney International*, **15**, 534–41.

Lalich, J.L. Burkholder, P.M. & Paik, W.C.W. (1975) Protein overload nephropathy in rats with unilateral nephropathy. *Archives of Pathology*, **99**, 72–9.

Leibetseder, J. & Neufeld, K. (1991) Dietary recommendation for dogs with chronic renal failure, p. 271. *Proceedings WSAVA XVI Congress*, Vienna, Austria.

Lewis, L.D., Morris, M.L. & Hand, M.S. (1987) *Small Animal Clinical Nutrition III.* Mark Morris Associates, Topeka, Kansas.

Maschio, G., Tessitore, N., D'Angelo, A. *et al.* (1980) Early dietary phosphorus restriction and calcium supplementation in the prevention of renal osteodystrophy. *American Journal of Clinical Nutrition*, **33**, 1546.

Massry, S.G. (1980) Requirements of Vitamin D metabolites in patients with renal disease. *American Journal of Clinical Nutrition*, **33**, 1530–5.

Mosier, J.E. (1988) *Proceedings of Symposium on Clinical Conditions in the Older Cat and Dog*, The Royal Garden Hotel, London, 15 June 1988, p. 5. Published by Hill's Pet Products Ltd, London.

Muller-Peddinghaus, R. & Trautwein, G. (1977) Spontaneous glomerulonephritis in dogs. *Veterinary Pathology*, **14**, 121–7.

Neugarten, J., Feiner, H., Schacht, R.G. & Baldwin, D.S. (1982) Ameliorative effect of dietary protein restriction on the course of nephrotoxic serum nephritis. *Clinical Research*, **30**, 54A (abstract).

NRC (1985) *Nutrient Requirements of Dogs*, revised edn. National Research Council, National Academy Press, Washington.

NRC (1986) *Nutrient Requirements of Cats*, revised edn., National Research Council, National Academy Press, Washington.

Oliver, J.E. (1987) Chapter 13 In: *Disorders of Micturition in Veterinary Neurology* (eds Oliver, Hoerlein and Meyhew). W.B. Saunders, Philadelphia.

Osborne, C.A. (1980) Symposium on polyuric renal disease in the dog. *Annual AVMA Meeting.*

Pitts, R.F. (1944) The effects of infusing glycine and of varying dietary protein intake on renal haemodynamics in the dog. *American Journal of Physiology*, **142**, 355–65.

Polzin, D.J. & Osborne, C.A. (1988) The importance of egg protein in reduced protein diets designed for dogs with renal failure. *Journal of Veterinary Internal Medicine*, **2**, 15–21.

Polzin, D.J. & Osborne, C.A. (1990) Prophylaxis of acute renal failure – strategies for avoiding renal disasters. *American Animal Hospital Association 57th Annual Meeting Proceedings*, pp. 441–5.

Polzin, D.J., Leininger, J. & Osborne, C.A. (1988) Development of renal lesions in dogs after 11/12 reduction of renal mass. Influence of dietary protein intake. *Laboratory Investigation*, **58**, 172–83.

Polzin, D.J., Osborne, C.A., Hayden, D.W. & Stevens, J.B. (1983) Effects of modified protein diets in dogs with chronic renal failure. *Journal of the American Veterinary Medical Association*, **183**, 980–6.

Polzin, D.J., Osborne, C.A., Hayden, D.W. & Stevens, J.B. (1984) Influence of reduced protein diets on morbidity and renal function in dogs with induced chronic renal failure. *American Journal of Veterinary Research*, **45**, 506–17.

Polzin, D.J., Osborne, C.A. & Lulich, J.P. (1991) Effects of dietary protein/phosphate restriction in normal dogs and dogs with chronic renal failure. *Journal of Small Animal Practice*, **32**, 289–95.

Proceedings of a Symposium on Canine Urinary Tract Problems (1989). SAVB-Flanders.

Ralston, S.L. & Fox, P.R. (1988) Dietary management, nutrition and the heart. In: *Canine and Feline Cardiology* (ed. P.R. Fox), pp. 219–28. Churchill Livingstone, Edinburgh.

Robertson, J.L., Goldschmidt, M., Kronfeld, D.S. *et al.* (1986) Long-term response to high dietary protein in dogs with 75% nephrectomy. *Kidney International*, **29**, 511–19.

Rocha, D.M., Faloona, G.R. & Unger, R.H. (1972) Glucagon stimulating activity of 20 amino acids in dogs. *Journal Clinical Investigation*, **51**, 2346–51.

Ross, L.A., Finco, D.R. & Crowell, W.A. (1982) Effect of dietary phosphorus restriction on the kidneys of cats with reduced renal mass. *American Journal of Veterinary Research*, **43**, 1023–6.

Rutherford, W.E., Bordier, P., Marie, P. *et al.* (1977) Phosphate control and 25-hydroxycholecalciferol administration in preventing experimental renal osteodystrophy in the dog. *Journal of Clinical Investigation*, **60**, 332–41.

Salusky, I., Kleinknecht, C., Broyer, M. & Gubler, M-C. (1981) Prolonged survival and stunting, with protein-deficient diets in experimental uraemia: reversal of these effects by addition of essential amino acids. *Journal of Laboratory and Clinical Medicine*, **97**, 21–30.

Schmidt, R.W., Bourgoigne, J.J. & Bricker, N.S. (1974) On the adaptation in sodium excretion in chronic uraemia. *Journal of Clinical Investigation*, **53**, 1736–41.

Shannon, J.A., Jolliffe, N., & Smith, H.W. (1932) The excretion of urine in the dog. IV The effect of maintenance diet, feeding etc. upon the quantity of glomerular filtrate. *American Journal of Physiology*, **101**, 625–38.

Stone, E.A., Littman, M.P., Robertson, J.L. & Bovee, K.C. (1988) Renal dysfunction in dogs with pyometra. *Journal of the American Veterinary Medical Association*, **193**, 457–64.

Walser, M. & Mitch, W. (1977) Dietary management of renal failure. *The Kidney*, **10**, 13.

Weiser, W.G., Spangler, W.L. & Gribble, D.H. (1971) Blood pressure measurement in the dog. *Journal of the American Veterinary Medical Association*, **171**, 364–368.

Chapter 6
NEOPLASIA IN OLD AGE

KEY POINTS

(1) Neoplasia is common in cats and dogs and should be considered in the differential diagnosis list of any geriatric animal presenting with non-specific signs such as weight loss, polydipsia, polyuria or recurrent signs such as pyrexia.

(2) Whenever possible avoid exposure to known risk factors.

(3) Vaccination against viruses that can cause cancer (e.g. feline leukaemia virus) should be widely practised.

(4) Early detection and treatment is desirable, so the regular screening of animals through middle age and old age is recommended.

(5) However benign a tumour looks – always biopsy neoplasms to obtain a definitive laboratory diagnosis.

(6) Surgery and chemotherapy can be employed successfully for the treatment of neoplasia – even in the most debilitated of old animals, but additional screening and supportive management may be necessary to avoid undesirable but predictable age-related complications.

(7) Nutritional support is important for the successful management of neoplasia in geriatric patients.

(8) Avoid breeding from animals with a high risk of developing neoplasia.

6.1   INTRODUCTION

Neoplasia is the uncontrolled multiplication of abnormal cells which do not respond to normal homeostatic controls and yet they are poorly recognised as being abnormal by the body's normal defence mechanisms. This allows them to proliferate, invade locally, undergo metastatic spread and ultimately cause clinical signs of disease or even death.

The key features of a neoplasm which differentiate it from other forms of cell growth are:

(1) excessive tissue growth
(2) unresponsive to normal control mechanisms
(3) not dependent upon initial stimulus to be present for continual growth.

Growth factors are the major regulators of mammalian cell growth in the body and they act via receptors on the cell surface. It is known that some genes which can induce the development of neoplasia (oncogenes), work through their action on growth factors (GF), GF receptors or proteins involved in transferring GF signals across the cell membrane (Slauson & Cooper 1990).

Neoplastic cells (particularly those in malignant tissue) are different from normal cells and *in vitro* demonstrate changes in biochemistry, antigenicity, karyotype and cell surface characteristics.

Neoplasms are classified as benign or malignant based upon their characteristics (see Table 6.1).

Table 6.1 Characteristics of benign and malignant neoplasms.

Characteristic	Benign	Malignant
Histological differentiation	Well differentiated – similar to originating tissue	Usually poorly differentiated
Invasion of adjacent tissue	Non-invasive. Often well circumscribed and capsulated	Invade adjacent tissues and cross tissue boundaries
Rate of growth	Slow	Rapid
Mitotic index	Low	High
Metastases	Never	Sometimes

Although there are some factors known to be associated with the development of neoplasia (see below) there is no single common biological mechanism that explains why cancer occurs and the initiation and progression of any specific neoplastic growth is influenced by many factors – most of which have still to be fully elucidated.

6.2 EPIDEMIOLOGICAL STUDIES

Neoplasia is common in cats and dogs but care is needed when interpreting studies which include statistical analyses relating to prevalence and incidence because for companion animals these studies often contain a relatively low number of animals, and invariably they have been conducted using the case load presented to second opinion referral centres and not those in first opinion practices, or in the population as a whole. Geographical variation in cancer incidence is also an important consideration when comparing reports from different parts of the world.

Dorn *et al.* (1968b) reported the annual incidence rate of neoplasia in dogs to be 381.2 per 100 000 population, and Priester & Mantel 1971 reported an annual incidence rate of 687 per 100 000 population. Between 34% (Dorn *et al.* 1968a) and 40% (Priester & Mantel 1971) were reported to be malignant neoplasms in dogs. It has been estimated that 50% of dogs aged over 10 years die of neoplasia (Kitchell 1988).

The estimated rate of occurrence for feline neoplasia is 264.3 per 100 000 (Hodgkins 1980).

The commonest neoplasms reported to occur in dogs and cats are shown in Tables 6.2 to 6.5. For tumours of the skin, for example, the mean age for almost all types of tumour is over 8 years, and only canine cutaneous histiocytoma and mast cell tumours are commonly seen in animals less than 5 years of age (Dobson and Gorman 1988).

Most of the papers published on the incidence of neoplasia are generated by academic institutions and are based upon referral cases. This presents us with a serious weakness in interpretation because common, easily rectified cases are dealt with by the first opinion practice and are not referred on. For example, testicular tumours, e.g. sertoli cell tumours are common in male dogs and yet they do not feature in Table 6.2.

After thyroid adenomas, lymphomas are the most common neoplasms in cats and advancing age is an important factor in some forms but not others.

Factors that are known to influence the occurrence of neoplasia are given in Table 6.6.

The majority of neoplasms occur in older dogs and the relative risk of neoplasia increases with age there being a peak occurrence at an average age of 8 years, however some neoplasms are also common in younger animals (Table 6.7). The precise relationship between advancing age and the occurrence of neoplasia has not been determined but with advancing time:

Table 6.2 Neoplasms in dogs.

Neoplasm	Association	Age a factor
Epithelial neoplasia	Account for approximately 48.3% of dog tumours*	Incidence increases in dogs over 5 years age†
Mesenchymal neoplasia	Account for approximately 24.6% of dog tumours*	Incidence increases in dogs over 7 years age†
Oropharyngeal neoplasia	Account for approximately 10.3% of dog tumours* Brachycephalic breeds	Incidence increases in dogs over 10 years age†
Skin neoplasia	Most frequent tumours in dogs (24–30%) of which 20% are malignant* Breeds at high risk: boxer, Boston terrier, Scottish terrier and others	Median age for cutaneous tumours in dogs is 10.5 years, and for cats 12 years
Mammary neoplasia	A common tumour in dogs (11.4%); 50% are malignant*. Over 97% of cases occur in females hence female sex hormone-related Entire females have 7 × risk of neutered females. Bitches neutered before first oestrus have 0.5 risk of those neutered afterwards	
Prostatic neoplasia	Male sex hormone-related	
Perianal adenoma	Male sex hormone-related Male dogs have 7.3 × risk of females	
Lipoma	More frequent in females than males Infiltrative lipoma occurred in dogs with a median age of 6 years and 87% of them weighed over 20 kg body weight More common in obese than non-obese animals	Aged dogs were labrador retrievers (Bergman *et al.* 1994)
Gastrointestinal tract neoplasia	Account for 15.1% of tumours in dogs, of which 50% are malignant*	
Haematolymphatic system neoplasia	Account for 10.9% of tumours in dogs, of which 90% are malignant German shepherd dogs increased risk for splenic haemangiosarcoma	Haemangiosarcoma was most common in dogs aged 8–13 years (Prymak *et al.* 1988)

Table 6.2 Continued.

Neoplasm	Association	Age a factor
Bone tumours – osteosarcoma	Large and giant breeds of dogs at high risk – usually appendicular skeleton, e.g. great Dane, Irish wolfhound, rottweiler, St Bernard, German shepherd dog	Common in younger animals as well as older dogs
Tonsillar carcinoma	Mainly occur in urban environments. ? Air pollution a factor (Cohen *et al*. 1964)	
Lung carcinoma	Mainly occurs in urban environments. ? Air pollution a factor (Brodey 1961; Brodey & Craig 1965)	
Bladder cancer	? Industrial pollution a factor (Hayes 1976)	
Mast cell tumours		Mean age 10.2 yrs

(* Theilen and Madewell 1987; † Dorn *et al*. 1968b)

(1) The likelihood of exposure to influencing factors increases.
(2) The duration of exposure to influencing factors present in the environment increases.
(3) The more time there has been for oncogenes to express themselves.

6.3 DIAGNOSIS

The diagnosis of neoplasia can be simple when a solid mass can be visualised or palpated, or when it can be identified on radiographic or ultrasound examination. But care is needed when considering the visual appearance of a tumour alone because appearances can be deceptive! An innocuous looking tumour of the skin could be a mast cell tumour, or a small black growth in the mouth could be a malignant melanoma, and fibrosarcomas along the gum margin of dogs often look benign (even under microscopic examination they can be misdiagnosed as fibromas) but they are in fact extremely invasive.

In all cases the diagnosis should be confirmed by the histopathological examination of a biopsy, or occasionally by the examination of fine needle aspirates or other techniques for obtaining neoplastic cells, e.g. impression smears.

In many cases the clinical signs associated with a neoplasm are non-

Table 6.3 Canine testicular tumours.

	Leydig cell	Sertoli cell	Seminoma
Frequency in descended testicles	40%	20%	40%
Frequency in undescended testicles	Rare	60%	40%
Mean age	11.2 years	9.7 years	10 years
Size	Benign adenomas – usually small and not noticed	Slow growing but can become quite large (especially if intra-abdominal)	Usually small
Other signs		Induces feminisation syndrome in male with: pendulous prepuce, atrophy of contralateral testicle and abnormal behaviour	Can get acute signs due to haemorrhage or necrosis – similar to torsion
Metastases	No	10–20% do	6–11% do
Diagnosis	Incidental finding usually Histopathology	Histopathology – fine needle aspirate cytology	Histopathology – fine needle aspirate cytology
Treatment	Castration – scrotal ablation is currently recommended by some authors	Chemotherapy to reduce metastases plus castration	Chemotherapy to reduce metastases plus castration
Prognosis	Good	Good unless disseminated	Good unless disseminated

specific and are due to systemic side-effects called paraneoplastic signs (Table 6.8). In geriatric patients it is important to evaluate the significance of such signs to rule out the possibility of the presence of a malignant or benign neoplasm.

6.4   TREATMENT

There are a wide variety of methods available for the treatment of neoplasia in dogs and cats and in geriatric patients it is advisable also to treat

Table 6.4 Neoplasms in cats.

Site	%	Cell type	%
Lymph node	31	Lymphoma and lymphocytic leukaemia (about 50% are associated with feline leukaemia virus)	38
Haemopoietic	16	Miscellaneous leukaemia	20
Skin	7	Squamous cell carcinoma	9
Mammary gland	5	Adenocarcinoma	9
Nose	3–4	Fibrosarcoma	4
Soft tissue	3–4	Reticulum cell sarcoma	3
Oral cavity	3–4	Carcinoma	3
Bone, joint	3	Adenoma	2–3
External ear	2	Mast cell tumour	1–2
Thyroid adenoma	Very common tumour in cats*	Osteosarcoma	1

* NB This table has been compiled after Hodgkins 1980, and was based on data that existed **before** the recognition of thyroid adenoma as a common cause of hyperthyroidism in middle aged to old cats (no cases having been reported in a cat less than 6 years of age).

Table 6.5 Lymphomas in cats: age distribution.

	Median age (years)
Peripheral lymphadenopathy	10
Alimentary lymphoma	11.5
Thymic lymphoma	3
Renal lymphoma	5.5
Miscellaneous lymphoma	6
All types	6

the effects of paraneoplastic syndrome. For example, hypercalcaemia is most often due to haematopoietic malignancy (myeloma and lymphoma) and rehydration followed by corticosteroids are indicated. Once the patient is stabilised specific treatment for the neoplasia can be commenced.

Conventional surgery

Surgical excision is the most effective method of treatment for most canine and feline neoplasms. Benign tumours should be removed completely by surgery, and early, poorly invasive malignant tumours can also be totally

Table 6.6 Factors known to be associated with the onset of cancer.

Factor	Neoplasm	Examples of known associations
Advancing age	Most tumours	Mean peak incidence occurs at 8 years of age
Genetic susceptibility	Osteosarcoma	Giant breeds of dog
It is now generally accepted that there is a genetic basis to neoplasia: purebreds are more susceptible than crossbred animals	Multiple primary neoplasia	The boxer especially mast cell tumours, lymphosarcoma, squamous cell carcinoma and osteosarcoma
Chemical carcinogens (or their metabolites), and UV radiation all cause DNA damage and are mutagenic	Intranasal tumours	Doliocephalic breeds, e.g. Shetland sheepdog, collie and German shepherd dog
	Malignant melanoma (skin)	Heavily pigmented breeds e.g. Scottish terrier, cocker spaniel
Sex hormone-related neoplasia	Female hormones (progesterone)	Mammary neoplasia
	Male hormones (testosterone)	Prostatic neoplasia Perianal adenoma
Parasitic	Oesophageal cancer	Spirocerca lupi in dogs
Viral	Lymphosarcoma or leukaemia	Cats – gastrointestinal tract neoplasia associated with feline leukaemia virus
	Papilloma	Self-limiting disease (usually seen as oral papillomatosis) in young puppies
	Fibrosarcoma	Cats – due to feline sarcoma viruses (FeSV) – associated with FeLV helper viruses
Environmental carcinogens	Ultraviolet light	Squamous cell carcinoma of the pinna in white cats
	Industrial pollutants:	
	• Asbestos	Mesothelioma in dogs
	• Air pollution	Tonsillar carcinoma in dogs Lung carcinoma in dogs ?Bladder cancer in dogs
	• Other	?Intranasal tumours in dogs
	Inhaled carcinogens	

Table 6.6 Continued

Factor	Neoplasm	Examples of known associations
Post-trauma	Osteosarcoma	At old fracture sites in dogs
Inorganic salts	Osteosarcoma – often mid-shaft	At fracture sites (dogs) in which metallic internal fixators have been left *in situ* for long periods of time
Radiation X-ray Radioactivity	Various carcinomas	

Table 6.7 Neoplasms that occur in young animals.

Neoplasms that occur in young animals	Comments
Histiocytoma	Self-limiting disease
Mast cell tumour	Cutaneous
Papilloma	Self-limiting disease associated with virus
Lymphoma	Association with FeLV in cats
Osteosarcoma	Especially in large and giant breeds of dog
Fibrosarcoma	

Table 6.8 Paraneoplastic signs in cancer.

Clinical sign	Neoplasm	Cause
Weight loss – cachexia	All types – particularly malignancies	Complex alterations in carbohydrate, lipid and protein metabolism. Inappetance or anorexia
Weakness, tremors, behaviour changes collapse, seizures coma	Insulinoma, liver tumours, lymphoma, large tumours, e.g. fibrosarcoma	Hypoglycaemia
Polydipsia, polyuria, cardiac arrhythmias, renal disease (nephrocalcinosis) vomiting, diarrhoea, loss of appetite	Lymphoma, multiple myeloma, perianal adenocarcinoma, secondary bone metastases, mammary carcinomas, parathyroid tumours	Hypercalcaemia
Reduced skin turgor. High PCV. Electrolyte imbalances	Any tumour	Dehydration

Table 6.8 Continued

Clinical sign	Neoplasm	Cause
Polyphagia, polydipsia, polyuria, hyperactivity, weight loss, dyspnoea, tachycardia, hypertrophic cardiomyopathy	Thyroid adenoma (cats), thyroid carcinoma (dogs)	Hyperthyroidism
Collapse. Haemorrhagic gastroenteritis	Mast cell tumour	Hyperhistaminaemia
Haemorrhagic gastroenteritis	Pancreatic tumour (gastrinoma)	Hypergastrinaemia
Acute blindness due to retinal detachment, renal failure, cardiac failure	Thyroid tumour, renal tumour, phaeochromocytoma	Hypertension
Bleeding, lethargy, pale mucous membranes, hypovolaemia	Any tumour – particularly haematopoietic, haemangiosarcoma, leukaemia	Anaemia, thrombocytopenia abnormal coagulation
Seizures, renal disease	Multiple myeloma, lymphoma, leukaemia	Hypergammaglobulinaemia
Polydipsia, polyuria	Adrenal tumour (Cushing's syndrome)	Hyperadrenocorticism
Reduced appetite	Brain tumour	Suppression of hypothalamic function
Unilateral reduced testicular size, pendulous prepuce, pancytopenia	Sertoli cell tumour	Excessive oestrogen production
Thrombotic infarcts, bleeding and diathesis	Any tumour but especially haematopoietic tumours, haemangiosarcoma, carcinoma, lymphosarcoma, granulocytic leukaemia	Disseminated intravascular coagulation (DIC)
Lameness, periosteal reaction	Any tumour mass in chest (primary or secondary, benign or malignant)	Hypertrophic osteopathy – cause unknown
Intermittent weakness and collapse on exercise	Thymoma	Myasthenia gravis

removed. Larger, invasive neoplasms can be debulked, allowing natural defence mechanisms or other treatment modalities such as cryotherapy, radiotherapy, hyperthermia or chemotherapy greater opportunity to be effective.

On rare occasions highly malignant neoplasms will metastasise during or immediately after surgery, hence careful planning of surgical technique is necessary to minimise the risk of metastasis. For example, ligate blood vessels leaving a tumour mass before manipulation or cutting. If possible exteriorise the neoplastic mass to isolate it from a body cavity or under-lying tissue and pack it off well to prevent inadvertent transfer of malignant cells into the body cavity or local tissues during surgery. Neoplastic tissues should always be handled gently to avoid release of potent substances such as histamine and heparin into the circulation.

When excising tumours try to assess the limits of abnormal tissue and add an extra margin to ensure that the whole of the neoplastic mass is excised. Remove local lymph nodes if they are involved, but leave them if they are not.

Before surgery it is important to screen the patient to ensure that it is capable of surviving the anaesthesia and surgical procedure and both anaesthesia and surgery time should be kept as short as possible. If major organ system disease is present the patient should be stabilised before surgery unless the neoplasm is life-threatening. For all but the most minor of benign tumours chest radiographs are essential to confirm that lung metastases are not present.

Surgically removed neoplastic tissue should always be submitted for histopathological examination to confirm the diagnosis.

Surgery is least successful by itself as a treatment for lymphomas (unless an isolated mass), leukaemia, oral carcinomas, bone tumours and feline mammary tumours (which are almost always malignant).

Cryosurgery

Cryosurgery is the application of freezing cold to destroy abnormal tissues and it offers several advantages over conventional surgery:

(1) minimal haemorrhage
(2) fibrous walls of vessels remain intact
(3) can be repeated without an accumulated effect
(4) may induce immunostimulation following the release of tumour anti-gens
(5) easy technique.

Disadvantages of cryosurgery include:

(1) slow healing
(2) scar formation
(3) depigmentation of skin and hair coat
(4) relative cost.

Cryosurgery works best for tissues in which the cells contain water. It is less successful for tissues with little water, e.g. containing keratin, warts.

It has been used successfully for superficial tumours on the head and neck and in the oral cavity, and the author has used it successfully for the treatment of prostatic carcinoma following debulking by conventional surgery.

Laser surgery

The application of lasers in veterinary surgery is a relatively recent innovation. However they have been successfully used for the treatment of intraocular and other tumours.

The main advantage of laser surgery is the precision of application that is possible using magnification techniques, as this minimises damage to adjacent normal tissues, particularly when access to a tumour is difficult or the adjacent tissues are sensitive and important for normal organ function to remain. The main disadvantage is the relatively high cost.

Hyperthermia

Hyperthermia has been used in the treatment of certain superficial and isolated tumours in dogs and cats but the early success rates reported have been disappointing. However, the technique continues to be used in human medicine – notably for the treatment of early diagnosed forms of throat cancer in which recent results have been very encouraging.

Radiotherapy

Although originally employed as a method of treatment in veterinary patients as early as 1906 by Dr R. Eberlein in the Berlin veterinary school, radiotherapy is still only available at some of the veterinary schools, and a few other institutions in the UK. For this reason no details about recommended radiation dose rates will be given as it is still a specialist field and should only be performed in experienced referral centres.

Whatever the method of delivery of the radiation (by irradiation from a beam of orthovoltage X-ray or cobalt-60 gamma rays; by the surgical implantation of radioactive implants (cobalt or caesium needles); by the use of strontium probes; or by the parenteral administration of a radio-active substance such as radioiodine) the clinical challenge of using radiotherapy is to deliver a therapeutic dose of radiation to the target site while minimising its delivery to normal tissues in order to avoid excessive damage to normal tissues.

Radiotherapy is indicated for tumours which are not amenable to surgery and it is most successful when applied to certain tissue types – notably rapidly dividing cells. Table 6.9 gives an outline of the sensitivity of different cell types to radiotherapy.

Table 6.9 Cell sensitivity to radiotherapy.

Most sensitive	Intermediate	Least sensitive
Germinal epithelium	Endothelium	Erythrocytes
Gametes	Fibroblasts	Nerve cells
Bone marrow precursors	Hepatic epithelium	Muscle cells
Mucosal linings	Renal epithelium	

Side-effects of radiotherapy are listed in Table 6.10 and these should be minimised by restricting the area of exposure of normal tissue as much as possible.

Table 6.10 Side-effects of radiotherapy.

Alopecia
Depigmentation
Desquamation
Mucositis
Necrosis

During therapy these changes can lead to serious gastrointestinal disorders but fortunately the most radiation-sensitive tissues (e.g. epithelial surfaces) are also the most rapid to heal.

Neoplasms that can be successfully treated using radiotherapy include:

- cutaneous squamous cell carcinoma
- oral squamous cell carcinoma
- localised lymphoma, e.g. mediastinal lymphoma
- fibrosarcoma

- solitary mast cell tumours (dogs – but not in cats in which mastocytoma is usually multifocal/systemic)
- thyroid adenoma (cats).

Chemotherapy

The use of cytotoxic (anticancer) drugs in isolation or in combination is an important, if relatively recent, addition to the armoury of treatments for neoplasia in cats and dogs. However these are potentially harmful agents and are best administered by experienced oncologists.

As with radiotherapy the clinical skill necessary for the successful use of these drugs is to deliver a therapeutic dose to the site of the cancer, and at the same time minimise side-effects due to normal tissues being affected by these non-selective drugs – which usually affect the growth or cell division phase of tissues. The most common complication is myelosuppression leading to leucopenia, increased risk of infection and sepsis.

Toxicity is the main limiting factor in the application of chemotherapy and for this reason combination therapy employing lower doses of drugs with different modes of action is usually preferred. Even with this approach multiple drug resistance can occur with some neoplasms.

In all cases the general physical condition of the animal must be good and pre-treatment screening for renal and hepatic impairment is essential. Providing there is no evidence of major organ disease the absolute age of an animal is less important, except in as much as it might limit the period of lifespan that can be expected following chemotherapy. Usually one should aim to provide an animal with a normal quality of life for a period of at least 6 months to 1 year to justify the use of this form of treatment.

White blood cell counts should be performed every 2–6 weeks during treatment with cytotoxic drugs as myelosuppression is their main side effect. If the white cell count falls below 3×10^9/litre the drug dose should be halved. If it falls below 2×10^9/litre the drug should be withheld.

Some of the drugs commonly used for chemotherapy in small animal veterinary medicine are listed below in more detail.

Vinca alkaloids

Vincristine/vinblastine
The vinca alkaloids vincristine and vinblastine are used for the management of cancer and immune-mediated diseases in cats and dogs. They have been most successful when used against lymphosarcoma and

haematopoietic neoplasms, mammary neoplasms in dogs, and some sarcomas. Vincristine has also been used for transmissible venereal tumour in dogs. Vinblastine has been used less often mainly for primary lymphoreticular tumours and disseminated mast cell tumours.

The dose rate of vincristine for dogs and cats is in the range:

0.025–0.05 mg/kg body weight, *or*
0.50 mg/m^2 body surface

The induction dose is usually 8 treatments at 14–21 day intervals.
The dose rate of vinblastine is:

2 mg/m^2 body surface *every* 7–14 days.

Both drugs are administered by slow intravenous infusion. Perivascular leakage should be avoided because they cause local irritation and necrosis, hence use of an i.v. catheter is preferred. They can also be given mixed with isotonic saline and administered over a 4–6-hour period.

Both drugs are metabolised by the liver and excreted via the bile into faeces, so normal liver function is necessary and should be evaluated before their administration.

Alkylating agents

These are widely used and interfere with DNA synthesis. Side-effects include myelosuppression, gametogenesis, alopecia and gastrointestinal irritation.

Renal toxicity has also been reported following administration of alkylating agents to old animals – especially to cats.

Cyclophosphamide

The active principal of cyclophosphamide is released by hepatic microsomal enzymes so do not use in old animals if there is evidence of hepatic insufficiency. It is contraindicated if the patient is anaemic (common in renal failure) as it causes further bone marrow suppression. Haemorrhagic cystitis is a serious side-effect which necessitates withdrawal of treatment with this drug.

Low dose rate:

50 mg/m^2 body surface orally on alternate days, *or* for the first 4 days of each second week.

High dose rate:

100–300 mg/m^2 orally *every* 21 days.

Cyclophosphamide is usually used in combination with vincristine or prednisone for the treatment of lymphoma (cats and dogs) or mammary adenocarcinoma. It has also been used for multiple myeloma.

Chlorambucil
Chlorambucil is the slowest acting of this group of drugs.

Dose
2–5 mg/m^2 body surface orally on alternate days.

Usually given in combination with vincristine or prednisone.
Used for the treatment of lymphosarcoma, chronic lymphatic leukaemia and multiple myeloma.

Melphalan

Dose
Induction   1–2 mg/m^2 on alternate days until plasma protein is normal,
                 or
                 1–2 mg/m^2 daily for 7–14 days

Used mainly for multiple myeloma and other lymphoproliferative diseases. Anorexia and vomiting may occur as well as myelosuppression.

Antitumour antibiotics

These drugs inhibit DNA synthesis

Doxorubicin
Is used in the treatment of lymphoproliferative and myeloproliferative diseases, various sarcomas, and mammary, prostatic and thyroid carcinomas.

Premedication with an antihistamine is needed to prevent tachy-dysrhythmias, anaphylaxis and collapse.

Dose
Dogs   slow i.v. injection 30 mg/m^2 every 3 weeks up to a maximum of
         240 mg/m^2

Cats   slow i.v. injection 20 mg/m^2 every 3–6 weeks

Side-effects include myelosuppression and myocardial damage leading to cardiomyopathy. It is excreted in bile and is contraindicated if hepatic insufficiency is present in the patient.

Other cytotoxic drugs

Cisplatin

Inhibits protein synthesis. Cisplatin has been used in veterinary patients for the treatment of osteosarcoma, soft tissue sarcoma and carcinomas.

Dose

Dogs   by i.v. infusion 50–100 mg/m^2 over 15 minutes. Repeat 4–6 times at 3–4 week intervals

Dogs should be fully hydrated and concomitant antiemetic and diuretic therapy are recommended.

Side-effects include nephrotoxicity, vomiting and myelosuppression. The risk of acute renal tubular necrosis is so great with this drug that **it should be used with extreme caution in ageing animals**, and it is contraindicated if renal impairment is present.

The use of cisplatin is contraindicated in cats.

Success of chemotherapy

Several forms of neoplasm have been treated successfully with chemotherapy and some current recommendations are listed in Table 6.11 (after Owen 1986).

Lymphosarcoma has been successfully managed using a combination of cyclophosphamide, vincristine and *L*-asparaginase.

Contrast the results of chemotherapy in Table 6.11 with those reported by Kitchell (1988) from the Universities of Ohio, Pennsylvania and UC Davis (Table 6.12).

Table 6.11 Success rates in chemotherapy (after Owen, 1986).

Success reported	*Type of neoplasia*
Successfully used	Lymphosarcoma Leukaemia Multiple myeloma Mastocytoma
Sometimes used	Soft tissue sarcomas Bladder carcinoma Thyroid tumours Mammary carcinomas Transmissible venereal tumour
Not very successful	Melanomas (oral) Osteosarcomas Haemangiosarcoma

Table 6.12 Success rates in chemotherapy (after Kitchell, 1988).

Tumour	Number	Response rate (%)
Haemangiosarcoma	9	100
Undifferentiated sarcoma	4	100
Neurofibrosarcoma, haemangiopericytoma, rhabdomyosarcoma and myxosarcoma	1 of each type	100
Carcinoma	7	86
Fibrosarcoma	9	33
Mesothelioma	1	0
Osteosarcoma	1	0

Immunomodulation

Prednisone

Corticosteroids such as prednisone are used widely in the treatment of neoplasia because they have antimitotic and cytolytic effects on lymphoid tissue as well as anti-inflammatory and immunomodulating effects. They are particularly useful for the treatment of lymphoproliferative disorders, mast cell tumours, and possibly brain tumours.

Dose
$10–60\,mg/m^2$ daily or on alternate days.

Side-effects can include pancreatitis and gastrointestinal upsets and with long term use suppression of adrenocortical function.

Nutrition

Cancer cachexia is very common even in patients maintaining normal food intake, indeed weight loss may be the first sign of the presence of a malignancy. In humans patients with cancer cachexia have reduced quality of life, are less responsive to treatment and have reduced survival times compared with similar patients maintaining body weight. The weight loss that occurs in cancer patients is due to a net energy deficiency resulting from inadequate intake, excessive energy expenditure or both. Possible factors include:

(1) **Reduced food intake:**

- altered taste or smell sensation
- intermediary metabolites acting on the satiety centre (e.g. serotonin)
- hepatic disease
- paraneoplastic syndrome – hypercalcaemia
- mechanical disorders – pain, tumour presence, post-treatment.

(2) **Hypermetabolism.** Increased metabolic rate resulting in increased rate of energy utilization.

(3) **Energy competition.** The neoplasm competes with the body for energy. It has been demonstrated that tumour cells preferentially metabolise glucose using anaerobic glycolysis, which is an energy wasting metabolic pathway, resulting in lactate production. The glucose used by the cancer is lost to the patient and the lactate produced is converted by the Cori cycle back to glucose, which further utilises energy. It has been estimated that the rate of turnover of glucose in cancer patients is 80% greater than in normal patients.

Dogs with lymphoma (before the development of cachexia) have increased lactate and insulin serum concentrations compared with control dogs and therefore they have significant alterations in carbohydrate metabolism (Vail *et al.* 1989). For this reason rehydration with glucose containing or lactated Ringer's solution should be avoided.

(4) **Impaired gastrointestinal function.** This may result in reduced digestion or absorption due to the physical presence of the tumour, a side-effect of treatment or paraneoplastic syndrome.

(5) **Impaired metabolic function.** Impaired metabolic function (e.g. haematopoietic, hepatic, renal or other) may result in impaired transportation, and metabolism of nutrients.

(6) **Paraneoplastic syndrome.** Many tumours induce metabolic changes which contribute to cachexia.

(7) **Excessive nutrient losses.** Losses may be caused by, e.g. gastrointestinal lymphosarcoma, haemorrhage, nephrotic syndrome.

(8) **Side-effects of cancer treatment.** These occur particularly with chemotherapy, radiotherapy and major surgery.

One consequence of cancer cachexia is negative nitrogen balance caused by protein degradation because the tumour uses amino acids for protein synthesis and for energy, at a rate which exceeds the patient's rate of protein synthesis. The resulting loss of lean body mass and protein depletion results in impaired immune function, reduced gastrointestinal function, hypoalbuminaemia and poor wound healing.

Several changes in lipid metabolism including a net depletion of lipid stores and hyperlipidaemia occur in cancer patients. The latter has been associated with immunosuppression and is possibly related to the poor survival times of some patients. Insulin resistance and sometimes insulin deficiency both develop in some cancer patients and this encourages fat mobilisation and leads to hyperglycaemia and poor glucose utilisation by the body cells, forcing them to use fat and protein for energy.

The mechanisms causing these metabolic changes have still to be fully elucidated, but it is known that they can occur before weight loss. Various factors including interferons and interleukons are probably involved as is the polypeptide tumour necrosis factor (also called cachectin) which causes lipid mobilisation, as does toxohormone, another tumour derived hormone.

So far therapeutic treatments alone have not proved successful at reversing cancer cachexia, and so whatever the underlying cause adequate and sometimes aggressive nutritional support should be provided for patients showing significant weight loss. Animals in a catabolic state are vulnerable to the side-effects of many of the treatment modalities that are recommended in the management of cancer, so stabilisation is recommended before commencing such treatment.

Feeding methods should be designed to:

(1) increase nutrient intake
(2) inhibit gluconeogensis and glycolysis
(3) prevent glucose utilisation by the cancer cells
(4) maintain nitrogen balance with amino acids
(5) provide branched-chain amino acids to decrease brain uptake of tryptophan and excess serotonin synthesis.

Diets containing 30–50% of calories as fat (which cannot be used as an energy source by cancer cells) have been shown to decrease glucose intolerance, fat loss and tumour growth and at the same time increase host weight, nitrogen and energy balance.

Whenever possible patients should be fed a high energy ration orally, but if voluntary food intake is inadequate nasogastric, pharyngostomy, oesophageal or gastric feeding should be employed. For debilitated cases a percutaneous endoscopically placed gastrostomy (PEG) tube is an easy procedure which is now routinely practised in many referral centres. Jejunostomy is another enteral route that can be utilised and, as a last resort, partial or total parenteral nutrition can be performed, but these techniques need to be carried out under the guidance of a trained clinical nutritionist.

There is some evidence that zinc supplementation might improve appetite and immune function in cancer patients and some authors recommend supplements.

Patients receiving nutritional support should be monitored regularly to assess progress. Body weight change and alterations in other parameters such as serum albumin, blood urea, red blood cell count and white blood cell count should be evaluated every 2 weeks.

Euthanasia

The method (or combination of methods) of treatment employed in a cancer patient must be based upon a critical clinical appraisal of the individual case; will depend upon the availability of different treatment protocols in the veterinary practice and, most importantly, should satisfy the wishes of the owner.

For many old people their pet is the main motivating factor that keeps them going and the prospect of losing their companion, particularly because of 'cancer' which is a very emotive subject, is hard for them to come to terms with. Communication about the diagnosis and case management needs to be dealt with in a caring and sensitive way.

Euthanasia is an important option to relieve suffering in cases in which the quality of life of the animal is unlikely to benefit from surgical or medical intervention.

Owners often require sympathetic counselling before, and following the euthanasia of their pet. This is particularly the case for owners for whom the pet is their last link with a member of the family who has left home, or who is deceased.

REFERENCES AND FURTHER READING

Bergman, P.J., Withrow, S.J., Straw, R.C. & Powers, B.E. (1994) *Journal of the American Veterinary Medical Association*, **205**, 322–4.

Brodey, R.S. (1961) A clinico-pathological study of 200 cases of oral and pharyngeal cancer in the dog. In: *The Newer Knowledge About Dogs*, pp. 5–11. Gaines Dog Research Centre, New York, NY.

Brodey, R.S. & Craig, P.H. (1965) Primary pulmonary neoplasms in the dog – A review of 29 cases. *Journal of the American Veterinary Medical Association*, **147**, 1628–43.

Cohen, D., Brodey, R.S. & Cohen, S.M. (1964) Epidemiological aspects of oral and pharyngeal neoplasms in the dog. *American Journal of Veterinary Research*, **25**, 1776–9.

Dobson, J.M. & Gorman, N.T. (1988) A clinical approach to the management of skin tumours in the dog and cat. *In Practice*, March, 55–68.

Dorn, C.R., Taylor, D.O.N., Frye, F.L. & Hibbard, H.H. (1968a) Survey of animal neoplasms in Almeda and Contra Costa Counties, California I. Methodology and description of cases. *Journal of the National Cancer Institute*, **40**, 295–305.

Dorn, C.R., Taylor, D.O.N., Schneider, R., Hibbard, H.H. & Klauber, M.R. (1968b) Survey of animal neoplasms in Almeda and Contra Costa Counties, California II. Cancer morbidity in dogs and cats from Almeda County. *Journal of the National Cancer Institute*, **40**, 307–18.

Hayes, H.M., Jr (1976) Canine bladder cancer: epidemiological features. *American Journal of Veterinary Epidemiology*, **104**, 673–7.

Hodgkins, E.M. (1980) Therapy of feline neoplasia. *Carnation Research Digest*, **16**(3), 1–4.

Kitchell, B.E. (1988) *Proceedings of Geriatric Medicine 1 Symposium.* Veterinary Post-Graduate Institute, Santa Cruz, California.

Owen, L.N. (1986) Cancer chemotherapy. *Veterinary Record*, **118**, 364–6.

Priester, W.A. & Mantel, N. (1971) Occurrence of tumours in domestic animals. Data from 12 United States and Canadian colleges of veterinary medicine. *Journal of the National Cancer Institute*, **47**, 1333–43.

Prymak, C., McKee, L.J., Goldshmidt, M.H. & Glickman, L.T. (1988) Epidemiologic, clinical, pathologic, and prognostic characteristics of splenic hemangiosarcoma and splenic hematoma in dogs: 217 cases (1985) *Journal of the American Veterinary Medical Association*, **193**(6), 706–12.

Slauson, D.O. & Cooper, B.J. (1990) Disorders of Cell Growth. In *Mechanisms of Disease*, 2nd edn., pp. 377–471. Williams & Wilkins, Baltimore.

Theilen, G.H. & Madewell, B.R. (eds) (1987) *Veterinary Cancer Medicine*, 2nd edn. Lea and Febiger, Philadelphia.

Vail, D.M., Ogilvie, G.K. & Wheeler, S.L. (1989) Alterations in carbohydrate metabolism in canine lymphoma. *Journal of Veterinary Internal Medicine*, **3**.

Chapter 7
NUTRITION IN OLDER ANIMALS

7.1 INTRODUCTION

Manipulation of dietary intake in older animals is necessary when there is either:

(1) frank clinical disease present
(2) subclinical disease present
(3) the nutritional requirements of the individual have changed.

Commercial pet foods have been formulated specifically for old dogs and in the future it is likely that foods will be developed for older cats as well. The justification for such products is based upon several premises:

(1) That older animals have different nutritional requirements from younger adults.
(2) That it is desirable to reduce the dietary intake of certain nutrients because they may be risk factors for the development, onset or progression of age-related changes.
(3) That it is desirable to reduce the dietary intake of certain nutrients because they may be risk factors for the development, onset or progression of disease processes.
(4) That it is desirable to increase the dietary intake of certain nutrients because of an increased requirement in older animals due to ageing changes in various organ systems.
(5) That it is desirable to increase the dietary intake of certain nutrients because of increased requirements due to the likely presence of subclinical disease.
(6) That many owners feed their animals a ration that greatly exceeds their nutritional needs.

Insufficient work has been done on the nutritional requirements of older cats and dogs or on the effects of nutrition on age-related changes, and so the first two premises are controversial. However, the role of certain nutrients in some common diseases of old animals is well documented and many of these diseases are often slow and insidious in their onset and progression, and so dietary manipulation may be beneficial. Good examples are endocardiosis in dogs (see Chapter 2) and chronic renal failure in both cats and dogs (see Chapter 5).

It is true that many owners feed rations that grossly exceed the nutritional needs of their animal so reducing dietary intake to meet requirements may be beneficial, will help reduce the likelihood of obesity occurring and is unlikely to be harmful.

7.2   AGE-RELATED CHANGES THAT MAY AFFECT NUTRITION

Age-related changes that may occur and affect nutrition include:

- reduced appetite
- reduced sense of taste
- reduced sense of smell
- reduced secretions – saliva, gastrointestinal secretions (including enzymes)
- reduced absorption?
- reduced transportation?
- reduced utilisation – liver
- reduced ability to excrete waste products – liver disease, renal disease
- increased requirement for nutrients – zinc?
- shift in body weight distribution from lean body mass to fat.

7.3   ENERGY

For any individual, energy requirements may stay the same, increase or decrease with advancing age. There are few studies looking at the energy needs of large numbers of old cats and dogs.

With advancing age a fall in basal metabolic rate has been recorded in humans and experimental animals. This is thought to be due to a change in the ratio between lean body mass and fat, there being an increasing tendency to lay down body fat with advancing age. There are several possible explanations for this trend:

(1) reduced thyroid hormone activity (secretion or receptor response)
(2) other hormonal effects, e.g. sex hormones, catecholamines.

Similar effects may also be seen in dogs and cats. Certainly there is an increased incidence of obesity in dogs with increasing age (Edney & Smith, 1986).

Energy requirements may also be reduced if an individual is doing less exercise due to changed behavioural patterns or secondary to other problems, e.g. an orthopaedic problem such as degenerative joint disease or osteoarthritis.

Older animals with reduced energy requirements should have their energy intake reduced otherwise obesity may result. Regular weighing of older animals should be recommended to detect any trend towards weight gain.

Obesity should be regarded as a serious problem in older cats and dogs. Obese animals have reduced glucose tolerance and hyperinsulinaemia (Mattheeuws *et al.* 1984a; Mattheeuws *et al.* 1984b) even in the absence of frank evidence of diabetes mellitus. Gross obesity can significantly reduce cardiovascular and respiratory function and also exacerbates numerous other problems such as skin disorders, and orthopaedic problems. Obesity in cats is a risk factor for the development of hepatic lipidosis and in cats and dogs it is a risk factor for the development of diabetes mellitus.

Most major organ system diseases seen in older animals (e.g. cardiac disease, renal disease, hepatic disease and neoplasia) result in catabolism and weight loss. This is particularly important in cats which, because of their high protein–calorie requirement rapidly break down their own body muscle and other available proteins in the presence of inadequate protein intake or excessive energy utilisation. Almost all chronic diseases in the cat result in significant weight loss or even cachexia.

When energy intake does not meet requirements additional energy should be provided and the selection of energy source (fat, protein or carbohydrates) will depend upon the underlying clinical status of the animal. In cats protein is a major provider of energy because of their obligate carnivorous nature, however fat provides 2.25 times more energy than either protein or carbohydrate and so this will often be the high energy source of choice for both cats and dogs. Carbohydrate will be used when high protein or fat intake is contraindicated in the individual because of the presence of impaired organ function or disease (e.g. renal failure, hyperlipidaemia).

7.4 PROTEIN

The protein requirements for geriatric cats and dogs have not been determined. In the absence of clinical or subclinical disease minimum protein requirements are probably the same as for adults. It must be remembered tht cats are obligate carnivores with higher protein requirements than dogs.

Protein intake should be maintained near to the minimum requirement in situations in which excessive protein intake is considered to be a risk factor for disease progression (e.g. chronic renal failure); or when excessive protein intake may have a direct clinical effect (e.g. hyper-ammonaemia in hepatic disease, and uraemia). It is controversial whether or not early dietary restriction of protein may prevent the onset of age-related progression of renal failure, though there is good experimental evidence that avoidance of excessive protein intake delays progression once renal damage is present (see Chapter 5).

It should be noted that no authorities recommend reducing protein intake below the minimum requirement, and that in the presence of chronic renal failure protein requirements may actually increase to twice that recommended for normal adult animals. Avoidance of unnecessary excesses is recommended not restriction below actual requirements. The term 'low protein' and 'protein restriction' which are in common use are therefore somewhat misleading.

Geriatric patients benefit from the feeding of high quality protein sources which are:

- highly digestible
- contain high concentrations of essential amino acids.

Protein sources with a high biological value include egg, liver and other animal source ingredients. Cereals have a lower biological value, but feeding a ration containing a mixture of plant and animal source materials can increase the overall biological value of the protein in the food by providing a better balance of amino acids.

7.5   FAT (OILS)

The fat requirement for old cats and dogs has not been determined and, in the absence of subclinical or clinical disease, it is likely to be the same as that for younger adults.

Fat is a high energy nutrient and excessive intake is likely to lead to the development of obesity, hence total daily intake should be controlled to maintain a fit healthy body weight.

Essential fatty acids have many important roles to play in the body including cell membrane structure and skin and hair coat condition. Some authorities consider supplementation of a ration with essential fatty acids of possible benefit for old animals, and it is unlikely to be detrimental unless excessive quantities are given in the absence of sufficient anti-oxidant in the ration (e.g. vitamin E).

Fat intake should be carefully controlled in the presence of liver disease, pancreatic disease, hypothyroidism and other causes of hyperlipidaemia. Cats and dogs rarely develop coronary artery disease and in these species dietary fat intake does not appear to be a risk factor for the development of cardiovascular disease.

7.6 CARBOHYDRATE

As long as the food contains sufficient quantities of gluconeogenic amino acids and fat, there is no dietary requirement for carbohydrate in cat or dog rations. However, in feeding trials carbohydrates in the form of starch are well utilised by both cats and dogs and it is a useful raw ingredient.

Carbohydrates in the form of dietary fibre may be beneficial in maintaining normal gastrointestinal function in geriatric patients because of their effects on motility and the water content of stools. They may decrease the occurrence of constipation in animals predisposed to develop it – though few clinical studies have been performed in the dog or cat. Fibre in the diet also reduces the bioavailability of all energy producing nutrients (i.e. fat, carbohydrate and protein) and so should probably be avoided in animals with compromised gastrointestinal function – particularly those with malabsorption.

7.7 VITAMINS

Some authors consider that older animals should be provided with increased quantities of vitamins in the ration to overcome reduced ability to digest and/or absorb them from the ration though there is little evidence to support this viewpoint.

Water soluble vitamins are lost from the body in the urine and polyuria such as accompanies chronic renal failure or diabetes are indications for increasing dietary intake to compensate for urinary losses.

Vitamin intake should probably also be encouraged in the presence of reduced liver function.

7.8 MINERALS

There is concern about the amounts of some minerals in rations fed to older animals, particularly:

Phosphorus

It is known that phosphorus retention occurs frequently in animals with chronic renal failure. This can result in calcification of various tissues including the kidneys themselves. For this reason high dietary intake of phosphorus should be avoided in older animals.

Controlling dietary phosphorus intake has been shown to delay the progression of renal failure in several studies (see Chapter 5).

Sodium

Many older dogs have endocardiosis which, even in compensated patients, results in sodium retention through activation of the renin–angiotensin–aldosterone pathway. Also, hypertension is a common problem in chronic renal failure in dogs and excess sodium load may make this worse. In humans clinically normal people with high salt intakes have higher blood pressure, and there is an age-related increase in blood pressure as well. Although primary hypertension is rare in cats and dogs some dogs are known to have salt-sensitive hypertension and recent studies at the Royal Veterinary College have demonstrated an increase in blood pressure with advancing age in cats and dogs (Bodey 1995 personal communication).

In the presence of congestive heart failure sodium intake should be minimised to decrease its effects on preload. While conventional treatment of dogs with endocardiosis states that treatment is unnecessary until heart failure is decompensated the author considers early introduction of reduced sodium diets helpful, particularly as the hypothalamic–pituitary–adrenal axis is stimulated early in the disease and switching old dogs from a relatively high sodium content ration to a relatively low sodium content ration can be difficult in some individuals due to acquired taste preference for salt (see Chapter 2).

Potassium

Potassium is very important as the main intracellular electrolyte in the body and depleted concentrations lead to weakness and neuromuscular abnormalities. Severe potassium loss can occur in renal disease leading to clinical hypokalaemia, therefore care is needed to avoid a ration with low potassium in such cases.

Zinc

Some authors suggest that older dogs require an increased dietary supply of zinc, presumably due to decreased ability to digest/absorb it. In cancer patients supplementation with zinc can lead to improved appetite and enhanced immune response.

Calcium

High concentrations of calcium in a ration can reduce the bioavailability of other minerals such as copper, zinc and phosphorus so excessive dietary intake should be avoided particularly in rations containing relatively small amounts of trace elements, and in individuals with impaired gastro-intestinal function such as malabsorption.

High calcium intake can also stimulate hypercalcitoninism and suppress parathyroid hormone activity which may be significant and complicate the clinical picture in some cases. Excessive calcium intake should be avoided as this can encourage the development of nephrocalcinosis and other soft tissue calcification in at-risk individuals.

REFERENCES AND FURTHER READING

Edney, A.T.B. & Smith, P.M. (1986) Study of obesity in dogs visiting veterinary practices in the United Kingdom. *Veterinary Record*, **118**, 391–6.

Mattheeuws, D., Rottiers, R., Kaneko, J.J. & Vermeulen, A. (1984a) Diabetes mellitus in dogs: relationship of obesity to glucose tolerance and insulin response. *American Journal of Veterinary Research*, **45**, 98–103.

Mattheeuws, D., Rottiers, R., Baeyens, D. & Vermeulen, A. (1984b) Glucose tolerance and insulin response in obese dogs. *Journal of the American Animal Hospital Association*, **20**, 287–93.

NRC (1985) *Nutrient Requirements of Dogs*, revised edn. National Academy of Sciences, Washington DC.

NRC (1986) *Nutrient Requirements of Cats*, revised edn. National Academy of Sciences, Washington DC.

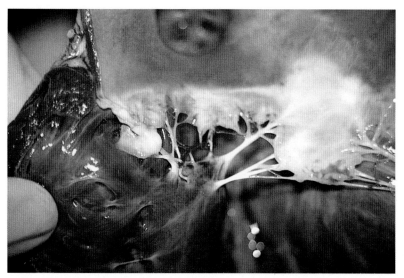

Plate 1 Endocardiosis lesions involving the atrioventricular valves of the heart are very common in ageing dogs. (Photo: A Boswood)

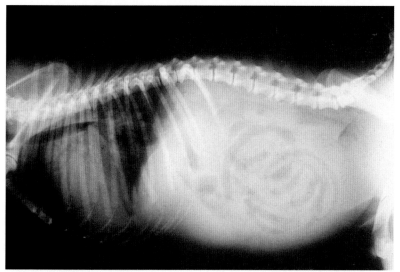

Plate 2 Radiograph of a seven-year-old terrier with exercise intolerance and a mitral murmur showing cardiac enlargement, dorsal elevation of the trachea, straightening of the caudal cardiac border, hepatomegaly, and abdominal distension with generalised 'ground glass' homogenous radiodensity obscuring soft tissue detail except for gas in the intestine lumen.
The radiograph also shows that this animal is in poor body condition – there is little muscle mass or fat over the dorsal spinous processes of the spine.

Nutritional support is needed and there is sufficient evidence on this radiograph to warrant full screening for renal and hepatic function prior to the administration of therapeutic agents.

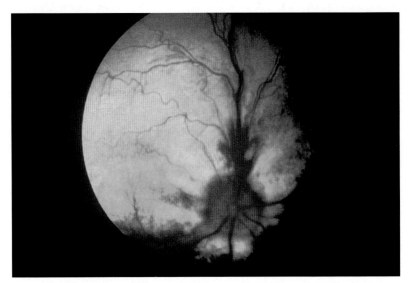

Plate 3 Ophthalmological examination of older animals may reveal the presence of retinal haemorrhages which are often bilateral. In such cases an underlying cause should be sought, e.g. hypertension secondary to renal disease.

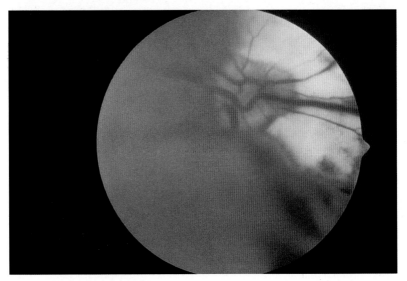

Plate 4 Retinal detachment can be acute or chronic and results in blindness. Sudden onset blindness may be due to bilateral retinal detachment which occurs secondary to the hypertension associated with renal failure.

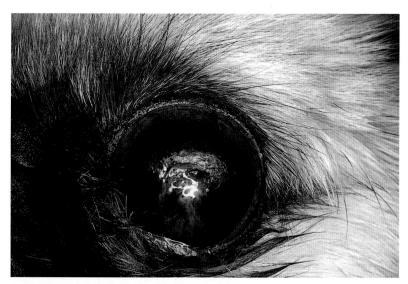

Plate 5 Chronic keratitis with ulceration and pigmentation.

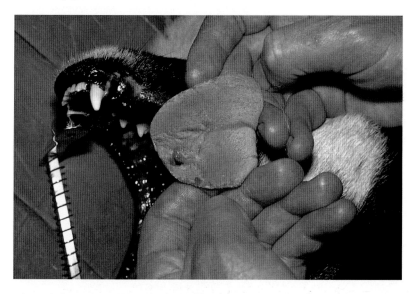

Plate 6 Squamous cell carcinoma of the tongue of a dog.

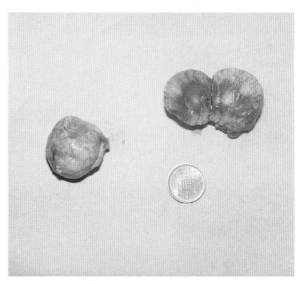

Plate 7 Chronic interstitial nephritis is common in old cats. The kidneys, like many organs in the body, have a large reserve capacity and are able to maintain function until over two-thirds of functional nephrons have been lost, as these grossly fibrosed and undersized kidneys demonstrate.

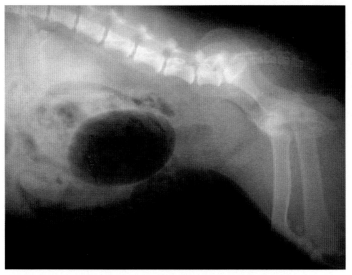

Plate 8 Contrast studies are necessary to diagnose prostatic enlargement, as in this dog with gross prostatic enlargement due to hypertrophy.

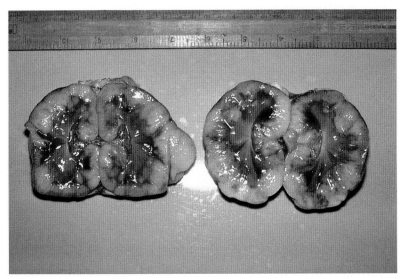

Plate 9 Renal lymphosarcoma is common in cats and may be associated with feline leukaemia virus infection.

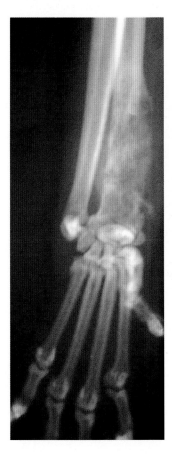

Plate 10 Twelve-year-old cat with neoplasia of the distal radius.

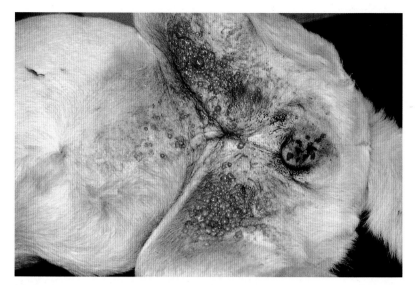

(a)

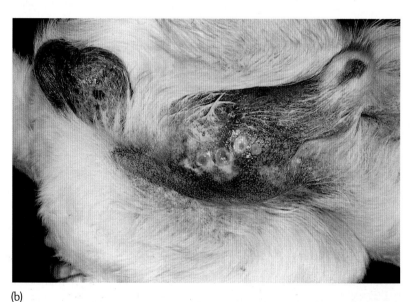

(b)

Plate 11 Differentiating between malignant neoplastic spread (**plate a**) and chronic infection (**plate b**) can be impossible from physical analysis alone, and biopsy and histopathological examination are necessary to confirm this diagnosis.

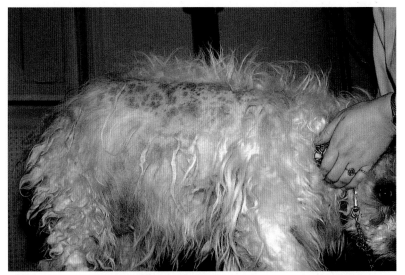

Plate 12 An eight-year-old West Highland terrier showing the typical external signs of bilateral alopecia and a pendulous abdomen associated with hyperadrenocortism.

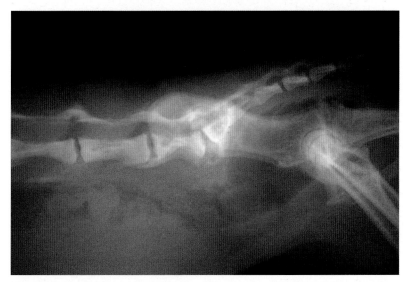

Plate 13 Spondylosis is common in older dogs, particularly at the lumbosacral junction as in this case. Such radiographic changes need to be differentiated from diskospondylitis and (rarely) from metastatic spread from local tumours (e.g. prostatic carcinoma).

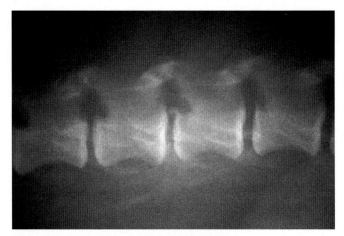

Plate 14 Disk prolapse in an old dog.

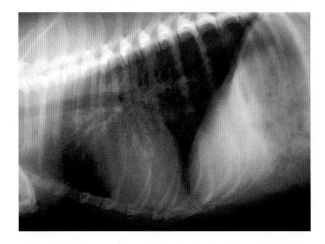

Plate 15
Lateral radiograph of the chest of an eight-year-old Jack Russell terrier showing chronic bronchial pattern with typical 'tramlines' 'doughnuts'.

Plate 16
An example of miliary secondary neoplastic spread to the chest. Metastases to the lungs is common in veterinary patients, and survey radiographs should be obtained before the treatment of primary tumours at remote sites is commenced.

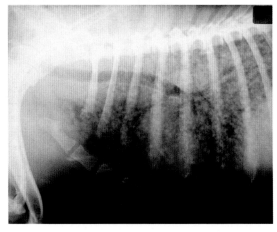

Chapter 8
ANAESTHESIA AND SURGERY IN GERIATRIC PATIENTS

KEY POINTS

(1) Advancing age is not in itself a contraindication to general anaesthesia or major surgery.

(2) Preoperative screening of old patients for the presence of sub-clinical disease or impaired organ function is necessary before anaesthesia or surgery.

(3) Anaesthetic doses should be based on lean body weight **not** actual body weight if the animal is obese.

(4) Generally, anaesthetic and other drug doses need to be reduced in ageing patients.

(5) Attempts must be made to avoid the development of hypothermia and hypotension during anaesthesia of old patients.

(6) Reduce exposure to known risk factors for acute organ failure, especially acute renal failure.

8.1 OBJECTIVES OF SURGERY IN OLD PATIENTS

The objective of performing surgery in geriatric patients is to prolong active, enjoyable life and procedures that offer no benefits to the patient should be avoided. However, a policy of avoiding all 'high risk' surgery would deny some patients with responsive conditions the benefits of surgical treatment.

The decision to perform elective surgery on old patients has to be a clinical judgement following full discussion with the owner. Owners should be made aware that older patients generally need preoperative screening, take longer to recover, require more post-surgical nursing, and may need careful (sometimes expensive) monitoring.

Ageing changes affecting the liver, kidneys, and the cardiovascular and respiratory systems are of major importance in anaesthesia. To maximise the benefits of any surgical procedure the physiological, pharmacological and pathological changes commonly seen in older animals need to be understood by both the surgeon and the anaesthetist.

A substantial proportion of surgery is performed in older animals, for example for the removal of tumours, and advancing age is not in itself a contraindication to major surgery or to the administration of a general anaesthetic. However, it is important to assess the elderly patient fully before surgery because they frequently have multiple organ system disease necessitating modifications in technique. Postoperative support is also very important, and mortality and morbidity may be higher if pre- and post-surgical risk factors are not managed properly.

8.2   AGE-RELATED TISSUE CHANGES THAT MAY AFFECT ANAESTHESIA OR SURGERY

Age-related changes that may affect anaesthesia or surgery include:

Nervous system

Central nervous system

Reduced functional tissue in the CNS is probably one of the factors that reduces the anaesthetic dose needed in older patients.

Old patients often have sluggish, impaired or absent reflex responses (e.g. pupillary light reflex) which may complicate monitoring during anaesthesia.

Loss of function of the special senses such as sight and hearing may lead to apprehension in strange environments (especially in cats), and some-times sedation is needed to reduce preoperative stress which otherwise can significantly increase sympathetic simulation.

Geriatric animals have reduced ability to generate body temperature and are susceptible to develop hypothermia, particularly during prolonged surgery or the postoperative recovery period. In this context it is important to remember that core body temperature may differ from peripheral measurements, and the use of oesophageal thermometers or infra-red thermometers (applied in the aural canal) may be preferable to rectal temperature recording.

Peripheral nervous system

Supersensitivity of postsynaptic receptors may prolong the action of muscle relaxants.

Interpretation of the significance of poor reflex responses during anaesthesia is more difficult in older patients than in the young.

Cardiovascular system

Subclinical and clinical cardiac disease is common in older dogs, and impaired cardiovascular function should be expected in elderly patients.

Baroreceptor function may be impaired, particularly in patients with chronic congestive heart failure, and the cardiovascular system's ability to compensate for surgical haemorrhage, or for the vasodilatory effects of anaesthetic agents may be inadequate resulting in severe hypotension.

Existing cardiovascular conditions such as congestive heart failure, cor pulmonale, sick sinus syndrome and the cardiac signs associated with hyperthyroidism in cats should be stabilised before general anaesthesia.

Anaesthetic agents depress cardiac function and cardiac arrest can be precipitated if cardiac arrhythmias are present, particularly ventricular arrhythmias that are refractory to therapy, right bundle branch block and bradycardia (heart rate below 60 in dogs; below 80 in cats).

Monitoring heart rate and systolic and diastolic blood pressures by direct or indirect methods is desirable throughout anaesthesia as is ECG recording, monitoring pulse character and regular examination of visible mucous membranes for capillary refill time.

Respiratory system

Age-related degenerative changes progressively decrease pulmonary function and physical changes occur in the lungs and chest wall. There is reduced alveolar surface area and diffusion capacity, pulmonary fibrosis, reduced lung elasticity, and reduced mechanical ventilation reserve. Chronic obstructive lung disease is common in old dogs and cats.

All of these changes impair gaseous exchange during anaesthesia hence oxygen supplementation is beneficial, and in some cases the use of bronchodilators may be indicated.

Impaired laryngeal function (sometimes laryngeal paralysis in older dogs – particularly Labrador retrievers) and increased respiratory dead space necessitate correct endotracheal intubation during anaesthesia and careful preparation of the patient to avoid vomiting. The use of antiemetic drugs (e.g. metoclopramide) might be indicated in patients requiring emergency surgical treatment, those with oesophageal or gastric motility problems or those with conditions likely to cause nausea (e.g. uraemia). A recent study suggests that older animals have a greater risk of developing gastro-oesophageal reflux during anaesthesia.

Pulmonary embolism is a common postoperative complication in old people, and may be more common than is currently appreciated in veterinary patients. In human general surgery patients the incidence of deep vein thrombosis is reported to be as high as 45% in those aged over 40, and 65% in patients over 71 (Consensus Conference 1986; Borow and Goldson 1981).

Renal

Impaired renal function prolongs the plasma half-life of drugs eliminated via the kidney and may alter fluid, electrolyte and acid–base balance, so screening for renal function is important before anaesthesia.

It is good practice to administer a balanced solution intravenously before and during anaesthesia to facilitate control of fluid, electrolyte and acid–base balance and to maintain renal perfusion. If renal hypotension occurs during anaesthesia tubular ischaemia may result leading to acute tubular necrosis and renal failure. Advancing age and general anaesthesia are both important risk factors for the development of acute renal failure. Other risk factors include the administration of non-steroidal anti-inflammatory drugs (NSAIDs), aminoglycosides, tetracyclines and other nephrotoxic drugs (Polzin 1991).

Liver

Most liver function tests usually remain normal in geriatric patients and this probably reflects the huge reserve capacity of this organ, however, in humans bromsulphalein (BSP) retention does increase with age.

Hepatic lipidosis is common in cats, and may or may not be associated with obesity. Up to 50% of liver biopsies taken from cats in the USA are reported to demonstrate lipidosis on histological examination (Davenport 1991 personal communication). This condition can be secondary to diabetes mellitus, hyperadrenocorticism, hypothyroidism or protein-energy malnutrition and affected animals may show gross hepatomegaly, elevated liver enzyme concentrations (serum alanine aminotransferase (ALT) and alkaline phosphatase (AP) and disturbances of liver function.

Cirrhosis is a chronic progressive disease usually affecting older animals resulting in loss of parenchymal mass and therefore reduced function. Primary and secondary hepatic neoplasia may also occur, eventually causing reduced liver function.

In the presence of impaired hepatic function the plasma clearance rate for drugs may be decreased resulting in increased duration of action. At the same time drugs and nutrients that need to be converted to an active form by the liver may exhibit reduced activity.

Endocrine

Thyroid

Serum T4 concentrations decrease by approximately 0.07 µg/100 ml per year in dogs with advancing age (Belshaw and Rijnbeck, 1979; Weller *et al.* 1983). If this fall has a significant effect thermoregulatory problems (hypothermia), and cardiovascular disturbances such as bradycardia or impaired myocardial contractility might be expected to result. Older animals might also be expected to have a reduced metabolic rate and a predisposition to develop obesity, which they do.

Hypothyroidism is relatively common in older dogs and may be associated with concurrent obesity. In some of these animals anaesthesia will be complicated by both the hypothyroidism and hypoinsulinaemia or insulin resistance. Hypothyroid animals are more susceptible to develop hypothermia and the vasodilatory effects of agents such as acepromazine and halothane may induce profound hypotension.

Adrenal

Aldosterone responses decrease in humans with advancing age and these changes are thought to be secondary to reduced renin secretion from the juxtaglomerular apparatus in the kidneys. In view of the high incidence of renal pathology in old animals it is reasonable to assume that such a decline might also occur in animals.

It has been suggested that corticosteroids should be administered to geriatric animals during prolonged periods of stress, surgery or anaesthesia to counter 'adrenal exhaustion'.

Hyperadrenocorticism (Cushing's syndrome) is most common in middle-aged to old dogs. It causes muscle weakness, reduced expiratory reserve volume, reduced chest wall compliance, increased blood volume and increased systolic and diastolic blood pressures (Feldman & Nelson 1987).

Adrenaline concentrations may increase, particularly in the presence of major organ system failure such as congestive heart failure. Plasma noradrenaline concentrations increase with age due to reduced clearance, but receptors compensate by becoming less sensitive.

Pancreas

Glucose tolerance deteriorates with advancing age and may be associated with hypoinsulinaemia (diabetes mellitus) or the development of peripheral insulin resistance. The administration of fluids containing glucose needs to be carefully considered in such patients, particularly if nutritional support is going to be given by total parenteral nutrition (TPN) when 50% dextrose solutions may be advocated. Chronic diabetics may have abnormal serum electrolyte concentrations which should be corrected before surgery.

In the presence of hyperinsulinaemia, hypoglycaemia may be precipitated during general anaesthesia and, as even a transient hypoglycaemia may cause brain damage, blood (and in some cases urine) glucose concentrations should be monitored during anaesthesia.

Obesity

In dogs the incidence of obesity increases with age. Obesity can impair cardiovascular, respiratory, hepatic and musculoskeletal function. Even in thin animals there is an increase in the body fat to lean body mass ratio with increasing age. When calculating the dose of an anaesthetic it is important to base it on the lean body weight – not on total body weight so some assessment of the degree of obesity is necessary. Large amounts of body fat alter drug pharmacokinetics.

Anaesthetic agents (being fat soluble) are taken up into body fat stores during prolonged administration such as intravenous infusion or during inhalation maintenance anaesthesia. These fat deposits act as a reservoir for the agent and prolong recovery time. The initial induction dose of short acting agents such as thiopentone sodium and methohexitone is not taken up into fat, but subsequent doses saturate skeletal muscle, and then are redistributed to fat. Repeated doses should be avoided in obese individuals.

Prolonged administration of halothane delays recovery because it has a high blood/fat solubility coefficient. On the other hand isoflurane is relatively insoluble in blood and fat and is probably more appropriate for use in obese old patients.

If the obesity is associated with hepatic lipidosis, drugs such as pentobarbitone which requires liver detoxification are probably best avoided.

Obesity may confound the identification of anatomical landmarks for the administration of local anaesthetic agents and it also increases the surgical risk of wound dehiscence and postoperative wound infection. Large amounts of perithoracic and intrathoracic fat may restrict chest wall excursion, lung inflation and compromise cardiac function.

Obesity sometimes occurs secondary to other conditions and this can present a diagnostic challenge to the clinician. Whenever possible uncomplicated primary obesity should be corrected by dietary management before elective surgery and anaesthesia.

8.3 DRUG–ANAESTHETIC INTERACTION

Many old animals are kept on long-term treatments such as non-steroidal anti-inflammatory drugs (NSAIDS), corticosteroids, diuretics, cardiac stimulants and anticonvulsants. A pre-surgical review of medications is important because they may affect anaesthesia.

Phenytoin and primidone are potentially hepatotoxic when they interact with anaesthetic agents and they also cause CNS depression, so reducing the dose of anaesthetic needed.

Chronic glucocorticoid administration may induce adrenal insufficiency predisposing to cardiac instability during anaesthesia. This is another reason why glucocorticoid administration immediately before induction of anaesthesia has been advocated.

Long-term diuretic administration may cause metabolic alkalosis, hypokalaemia, and sometimes hypomagnesaemia – all of which should be corrected before surgery.

8.4 PRE-ANAESTHESIA CHECK

It is important to review the presenting history in detail, perform a comprehensive physical examination and perform laboratory screening tests of geriatric animals for signs of subclinical disease or impaired organ function.

The author advocates the following as a **minimum** pre-surgery screening programme for geriatric patients:

(1) complete blood count and differential
(2) haematocrit
(3) total serum protein
(4) serum urea
(5) serum creatinine
(6) serum electrolytes (sodium, potassium, chlorine and calcium)
(7) blood glucose
(8) serum bile acids
(9) ECG examination
(10) urinalysis – protein, pH, glucose and sediment.

In an ideal situation the following would also be included in a geriatric screen:

(1) T4
(2) serum ALT, AP
(3) survey chest and abdominal radiographs
(4) arterial and venous blood gas analysis
(5) systolic and diastolic blood pressure measurement.

It is important to review recent medications and existing diagnostic information such as previous radiographs, or laboratory data.

8.5   LOCAL ANAESTHESIA

Local or regional anaesthesia may be safer than general anaesthesia in severely debilitated animals. Sedation is usually required, and perineural injection, field block, surface analgesia, intravenous regional analgesia or epidural and spinal injections can be used. Identification of anatomical landmarks may be difficult in obese subjects.

Epidural anaesthesia is a useful procedure when the anaesthetic is injected at the lumbosacral junction but cranial epidural should be avoided because sympathetic fibres may be blocked causing hypotension.

Acupuncture has been recommended as a method of providing analgesia for minor procedures in 'high risk' geriatric veterinary patients (Janssens *et al.* 1988).

8.6   GENERAL ANAESTHESIA

Preparation

Animals should be fasted for 12 hours, with water being withdrawn 1–2 hours beforehand. Water deprivation in old animals can precipitate a uraemic crisis so overnight deprivation is not recommended if there is evidence of renal incompetence and an i.v. fluid line should be established before the administration of a sedative or anaesthetic.

All patients should be weighed before computation of drug dosages to avoid errors. If the animal is obese the lean body weight should be estimated.

Premedication

Acepromazine can be given in low doses (0.025–0.05 mg/kg i.m.) but should not be used in the presence of cardiovascular disease such as endocardiosis and congestive heart failure, as it can cause rapid hypotension. Acepromazine should also be avoided in dogs prone to seizures, and it is contraindicated in the presence of renal impairment. Intravenous administration can cause profound hypotension and it should only be used by this route with great care. The author has witnessed a geriatric dog collapsing and dying immediately following the intravenous administration of acepromazine.

Xylazine and medetomidine should only be used with extreme care in geriatric canine and feline patients because they can cause deep and prolonged sedation with bradycardia and severe cardiovascular depression. Vomiting often follows their administration and this could result in aspiration in old animals with impaired laryngeal reflexes. Caution is needed when using these substances in the presence of pulmonary disease.

In dogs neuroleptanalgesics have the advantage that the narcotic component can be reversed by an antagonist. However they have profound effects on the cardiovascular and respiratory systems causing tachycardia or bradycardia, hypertension or hypotension, depressed respiration and cyanosis. After reversal some dogs relapse into a sedated state that may last for up to 36 hours.

These agents are contraindicated in the presence of impaired hepatic or renal function, should only be used at reduced dose rates (50% that recommended for adults) and with great care in elderly patients. When using narcotic analgesics or neuroleptanalgesics dogs should be premedicated with anticholinergics to avoid secondary bradycardia.

Induction

Inhalation can be used, but may induce excitation if the animal is not sedated and the associated catecholamine release can cause cardiac disturbances. Isoflurane has advantages over halothane because it is relatively insoluble in blood, causes rapid induction and does not potentiate the effects of adrenaline on the heart.

Some old animals, particularly those with catabolic diseases such as chronic heart failure, hyperthyroidism, sepsis and cancer may have a fall in body fat content with a concurrent decrease in body muscle mass and these changes can influence the distribution of i.v. anaesthetic agents increasing their efficacy and prolonging their duration of action. Reduced hepatic function may also prolong their duration of action and delay recovery. In general, intravenous anaesthetic doses should be reduced in elderly patients.

Older animals should be given only 50% of the dose of thiopentone sodium required by young adults, i.e. give 2–3 mg/kg i.v. over 10 seconds followed by small incremental doses given to effect over about 1 minute. A 2.5% solution is suitable for healthy, large dogs, but a 1.25% solution is recommended for cats, small dogs and debilitated cases. Give just sufficient to induce narcosis then mask/intubate. Premedication may be needed to reduce excitation during induction and recovery. Thiopentone is not good for anaesthetic maintenance because of tissue saturation and the prolonged recovery period that results. Concurrent administration of chloramphenicol, streptomycin or kanamycin can also prolong the recovery period.

Greyhounds and other dogs with little body fat may take 24 hours to recover from the effects of thiopentone, and methohexitone or propofol may be more appropriate. Methohexitone is shorter acting and the recovery period less than with thiopentone but it needs to be used with care as it can cause severe respiratory depression if administered too rapidly, and greater excitement or inadequate relaxation if administered too slowly.

Propofol has an action similar to thiopentone and it has the advantage that it can be used without premedication, but it does cause slightly greater cardiovascular depression. It has a less cumulative effect than thiopentone resulting in a more rapid recovery.

Pentobarbitone is rarely used in clinical practice nowadays. It is metabolised slowly and may cause profound respiratory depression. It is contraindicated in the presence of hepatic impairment and recovery time is prolonged with hypothermia being a postoperative complication.

Alphadolone and alphaxalone combination is commonly used to provide anaesthesia in cats. Some cats may develop respiratory embarrassment following rapid induction and the presence of underlying lung pathology may predispose to this. Slow administration of the anaesthetic is recommended to minimise the occurrence of such incidents.

Ketamine can be used as a sole anaesthetic in the cat, but in dogs it should only be used following premedication with xylazine. When used by itself muscle relaxation is poor, necessitating the administration of xylazine or a benzodiazepine such as diazepam. In cats vomiting often occurs during induction, and recovery from ketamine/xylazine anaesthesia can be prolonged for up to 8 hours in the presence of hypothermia. Xylazine also induces bradycardia and the administration of atropine immediately after the xylazine injection is recommended to counter this effect.

Induction with ketamine following premedication with acepromazine and subsequent maintenance with halothane or nitrous oxide alone or in combination has been recommended for cats with hyperthyroidism (Thoday 1990).

Respiratory depression is a consequence of all forms of anaesthesia and preoxygenation for 2–3 minutes before and during induction will help to prevent hypoxaemia.

The animal should be fully intubated following induction, to avoid excessive dead space.

Maintenance

Inhalation anaesthetics are preferred to intravenous drugs for maintenance anaesthesia in geriatric patients because most of the agent is excreted unchanged via the lungs and recovery is not dependent upon drug metabolism.

Intermittent positive pressure ventilation (ventilator or manual) has advantages during prolonged surgery in the elderly to facilitate the maintenance of blood gases within normal limits. It also saves the patient's body 'work', and offers a method for hastening the removal of anaesthetic agent in the presence of an overdose.

All general anaesthetics cause respiratory depression, and some impairment of respiratory function is likely to be present in this group of patients so oxygen flow rate should be maintained at 30–33% of inspired gas.

The most commonly used inhalation agents in small animal practice (halothane and isoflurane) can rapidly cause severe cardiovascular and respiratory depression if high concentrations are given. For this reason they should only be used with vaporizers specifically designed to be used with them. Isoflurane is preferred to halothane in old patients, because it does not potentiate the cardiovascular effects of catecholamines, cardiac output is well maintained at anaesthetic doses and it does not alter myocardial contractility, however it does cause a fall in total peripheral resistance which can precipitate hypotension.

Recovery is prolonged with methoxyflurane, and it is contraindicated in the presence of renal or hepatic impairment. Nitrous oxide does not alter blood pressure by itself and helps reduce the dose of other inhalation agents. It should be avoided in patients with severe respiratory problems preoperatively, or if hypoxaemia develops during surgery.

If muscle relaxation is needed during surgery administration of a muscle relaxant is preferred to increasing the depth of anaesthesia. Non-depolarising relaxants must be reversed by an anticholinesterase so atropine is given first to block the unwanted muscarinic effects (such as bradycardia) of the reversal agent.

Pancuronium is a medium-duration relaxant (lasting 30–45 minutes). It may cause tachycardia in cats and dogs and is contraindicated in the presence of hepatic or renal impairment and obesity. Vecuronium causes minimal cardiovascular effects and has a duration of action of about 30 minutes. Atracurium has a similar duration of action, also has minimal vagolytic or sympatholytic properties and it can be administered to animals with hepatic or renal failure.

Depolarising muscle relaxants are easier to use as they don't need to be reversed. In dogs suxamethonium at a dose rate of 0.3 mg/kg given intravenously will provide complete paralysis for 20 minutes. Supplements of 0.1 mg/kg can be given to prolong its effects. It is contraindicated in the presence of hepatic impairment. In cats 1.5 mg/kg produces paralysis for 5 minutes.

Supportive therapy

Intravenous fluids should be administered throughout anaesthesia at a rate of 10 ml/kg per hour. The rate should be reduced in animals with congestive heart failure or anuric renal failure, and monitoring central venous pressure is advisable. Urine output should be maintained at more than 0.3 ml/kg per hour in the dog.

The need for nutritional support of patients with catabolic disease is becoming increasingly important. Anorectic animals or those with recognised catabolic disease such as congestive heart failure or cancer, should be provided with adequate nutrition before elective surgery either by force feeding or tube feeding. Nasogastric tubes (Fr6) can be passed easily in conscious dogs and cats, and they offer a simple, effective way of providing nourishment to geriatric patients.

In some cases postoperative malnutrition can be predicted, and early placement of nasogastric (or naso-oesophageal), pharyngostomy, gastrostomy or jejunostomy tubes is advantageous. Diets for tube feeding should be high in energy density, provide adequate nitrogen in the form of protein, and be administered in a liquid formulation to facilitate passage down the tube.

Use of a heated pad, circulating hot water blanket or insulated blankets help minimise heat loss and prevent the development of hypothermia during anaesthesia. A fall in body temperature can greatly prolong the recovery period.

Monitoring

Throughout anaesthesia it has been recommended that the following parameters should be monitored (Dodman *et al.* 1984):

(1) heart rate and rhythm
(2) respiratory rate and character
(3) pulse rate and quality
(4) mucous membrane colour
(5) capillary filling rate
(6) ECG
(7) rectal temperature.

In some cases the following should also be monitored:

(1) arterial blood pressure (direct or indirect)
(2) urinary output
(3) haematocrit
(4) total serum protein
(5) blood gases.

Recovery

During recovery the environmental temperature should be kept warm, and fluid therapy and oxygen administration should be continued until the animal is conscious.

Endotracheal tubes should only be removed once laryngeal reflexes have returned. Antiemetic drugs may be indicated in patients exhibiting nausea or retching.

8.7 SURGICAL COMPLICATIONS

With increasing age skin loses its elasticity and vascularity making it vulnerable to trauma and it bruises easily. Gentle handling during surgery is therefore advisable.

Wound healing may be delayed in older patients, and there may be a reduction or delayed response in the formation of granulation tissue. Wounds in older patients may also be more susceptible to infection and patients with evidence of systemic infection, renal disease, hepatic disease, cardiovascular disease or endocrine disorders are likely to exhibit delayed wound healing.

Hypoproteinaemia will adversely affect wound healing by impairing fibroplasia, neovascularisation, remodelling and tensile strength so prolonging the healing phase. Maintaining a positive protein-energy balance in patients before elective surgery and during the postoperative recovery period is an important therapeutic objective which might necessitate special feeding techniques in some individuals.

Haemostasis needs to be vigilant during surgery because local blood losses may seem small if the patient has transient hypotension but could result in significant postoperative haemorrhage following recovery. Haemorrhage at wound sites is a major risk factor for the development of infection or dehiscence.

Advancing age, prolonged anaesthesia and surgery time, hypotension, obesity, some therapeutic agents and the presence of concurrent disease may all increase the risk of wound infection. The presence of gross obesity may delay return to normal mobility.

REFERENCES AND FURTHER READING

Belshaw, B.F. & Rijnbeck, A. (1979) Radioimmunassay of plasma T4 and T3 in the diagnosis of primary hypothyroidism in dogs. *Journal of the American Animal Hospital Association*, **15**, 17–23.

Borow, M. & Goldson, H. (1981) Post-operative venous thrombosis. Evaluation of five methods of treatment. *American Journal of Surgery*, **141**, 245–51.

Consensus Conference (1986) Prevention of venous thrombosis and pulmonary embolism. *Journal of the American Medical Association*, **256**, 744–9.

Cummings, B.J., Honsberger, P.E., Afagh, A.J. et al. (1993) Cognitive function and Alzheimer's-like pathology in the aged canine. II. Neuropathology. *Neurobiology of Aging*, **14**, 547.

Dodman, N.H., Seeler, D.C. & Court, M.H. (1984) Aging changes in the geriatric dog and their impact on anaesthesia. *Compendium on Continuing Education*, **6**(12), 1106–12.

Feldman, E.C. & Nelson, R.W. (eds) (1987) Hyperadrenocorticism. In: *Canine and Feline Endocrinology and Reproduction*, p. 137. W.B. Saunders, Philadelphia.

Janssens, L.A.A., Rogers, P.A.M. & Schoen, A.M. (1988) Acupuncture analgesia: A review. *Veterinary Record*, **122**, 355–8.

Morys et al. (1994) *NeuroReport*, **5**, 1825.

Polzin, D.J. (1991) Strategies for preventing acute renal failure. *Eastern States Veterinary Conference Proceedings Manual*, pp. 322–4.

Thoday, K.L. (1990) The thyroid gland. In: *Manual of Small Animal Endocrinology* (ed. M. Hutchison), pp. 25–57. BSAVA Publications, Cheltenham.

Weller, R.E., Kinnas, T.C. & Stevens, D. (1983) Basal serum thyroxine concentration and its response to thyroid-stimulating hormone administration decreases with chronological age in Beagle dogs. *Scientific proceedings*. American College of Veterinary Internal Medicine, New York, p. 38.

Chapter 9
RADIOLOGY IN GERIATRIC PATIENTS

9.1 INTRODUCTION

Radiology is an important aid to diagnosis in geriatric patients. It can help in the early detection of problems before clinical signs are evident and it can help in devising a plan for the management of a case. For example, all animals with neoplasia should be radiographed for evidence of secondary spread to the lungs or other vital structures before surgical attempts at removal. Care is needed not to overinterpret radiographic findings – for example it is dangerous to consider intrathoracic masses as being secondary metastases simply because a previous neoplasm was removed at an earlier date.

The ability of older animals to mask the effects of subclinical disease processes in major organ systems by compensatory physiological mechanisms that maintain homeostasis makes diagnosis and evaluation of such individuals a challenge. Evaluation of the whole animal is particularly important before an elective stressful procedure such as a surgical procedure under general anaesthesia.

Ageing changes occur in various organs and can present as unusual radiographic appearances to unsuspecting clinicians.

9.2 SKELETAL CHANGES

Ossification of the costochondral junctions gives an irregular radiodense pattern which may be mistaken for neoplasia or osteomyelitis.

Spondylosis is benign new bone development bridging adjacent vertebrae in the spine and it is particularly common in some breeds such as brachycephalics. The new bone deposition is usually smooth and of little consequence unless it entraps spinal nerves as they leave the spinal column. Spondylosis is particularly common at the lumbosacral junction and at this site a single lesion needs to be differentiated from discospondylitis which may also occur in older animals. In the latter cases there are clinical signs of pain, pyrexia and sometimes neurological deficits, and on radiography there is usually narrowing of the joint space, loss of bone in adjacent vertebral endplates, and sclerosis either side of the joint space as well as ventral (and lateral on dorsoventral projections) new bone bridging between the vertebrae.

Demineralisation of bone occurs in renal secondary hyperparathyroidism often before owners report the clinical signs such as polydipsia and polyuria associated with the underlying renal disease. Poorly mineralised bones with thin cortices are seen on survey radiographs, and the mandible is one of the first bones to be affected with teeth on radiographs of affected animals appearing to 'float' in the poorly radiodense bone.

Chronic, smooth spurs of new bone and smooth surfaced osteophytes may develop around joints (particularly on the distal femur and proximal tibia of the stifle, and at the interphalangeal joints) and they may be of no clinical significance. They need to be differentiated from the more aggressive new bone deposition associated with degenerative joint disease or osteoarthritis. It is useful to radiograph the contralateral joint to compare unusual benign appearances on radiographs. If the radiographic appearance is the same in both limbs it is unlikely to be directly related to unilateral clinical signs such as lameness.

9.3   SOFT TISSUE CHANGES

Survey radiographs can give a good indication of the nutritional status of an animal. Lack of fat over the dorsal spinous processes of the spine, and poor soft tissue detail (due to lack of mesenteric fat) on lateral abdominal radiographs both may indicate poor body condition.

Large deposits of fat over the spine, in the region of the falciform ligament in the cranioventral abdomen or around the apex of the heart may all suggest the presence of overnutrition or obesity.

Soft tissue organs should be examined on survey radiographs for changes in shape, contour, size, position or radiodensity.

In ageing animals several changes are commonly seen on survey radiographs which may have little or no clinical significance:

(1) In the chest cardiac enlargement (left sided, right sided or both) may occur in dogs in the absence of any clinical signs but associated with compensatory mechanisms such as in response to the leaking atrioventricular valves which occurs in endocardiosis.

(2) Many older dogs (particularly the brachycephalic breeds) develop a pronounced bronchial pattern (doughnuts and tramlines) on lateral radiographs of the chest due to thickening and calcification of the bronchial walls. These changes may or may not be associated with respiratory signs such as abnormal respiratory sounds on auscultation.

(3) In the abdomen hepatic enlargement is frequently noticed in both cats and dogs with the left hepatic lobe extending well beyond the costal arch on lateral views of the abdomen. Occasionally the liver size is reduced on survey radiographs, sometimes with cranial displacement of the axis of the stomach even though routine biochemistry tests for liver damage are normal.

(4) Kidney size may be reduced in the presence of progressive renal disease such as chronic interstitial nephritis in cats and increased in cases of renal hypertrophy or neoplasia, and the renal contour may be irregular due to fibrosis or the presence of neoplasia such as lymphosarcoma (which is also common in cats).

(5) Dystrophic calcification can occur in many soft tissues notably the kidneys (where it usually occurs at the junction between the cortex and medulla), heart wall, urinary bladder, prostate, tendons and skin. In tendons the likely cause is chronic inflammation due to repeated trauma. However, in all such cases a primary underlying cause such as hypercalcaemia due to paraneoplastic syndrome, or Cushing's syndrome should be sought.

(6) Animals with Cushing's syndrome (hyperadrenocorticism) and other conditions may develop calcification of the skin which, when overlying other structures, may confuse unsuspecting clinicians trying to interpret radiographs.

Interpretation of the significance of radiographic signs can be difficult in older animals. It is helpful if comparisons can be made with survey radiographs taken earlier in life to determine significant changes and, if sequential films are available, they will give an idea of the timescale of progression of a lesion. This type of information can be very helpful with the development of subtle changes in, for example, the lungs.

If it were not for the potential health hazards associated with obtaining good radiographic images, and for the need to administer a general anaesthetic to most animals to get them, a good case could be put for obtaining screening films at various stages of an animal's life. In future the use of safe, non-invasive imaging techniques such as ultrasound will undoubtedly add a new dimension to our ability to detect early changes in organs through routine screening examinations.

REFERENCES AND FURTHER READING

Douglas, S.W., Herrtage, M.E. & Williamson, H.D. (1987) *Principles of Veterinary Radiography.* Baillière Tindall, Eastbourne.

Kealy, J.K. (1986) *Diagnostic Radiology of the Dog and Cat,* 2nd edn. W.B. Saunders, Philadelphia.

O'Brien, T.R. (1978) *Radiographic Diagnosis of Abnormal Disorders in the Dog and Cat.* W.B. Saunders, Philadelphia.

Owens, J.M. (1982) *Radiographic Interpretation for the Small Animal Clinician.* Ralston Purina Company, Saint Louis.

Chapter 10
GERIATRIC SCREENING PROGRAMMES

10.1 WHY SCREEN GERIATRIC PATIENTS?

Over one-third of cats and dogs presented to veterinary practices are aged 7 years or over (SAPTU, demographic data supplied by the Small Animal Practice Teaching Unit, University of Edinburgh, August 1991) and there is a great deal of interest in this group of animals because of:

(1) the effect of ageing on major body system function
(2) the likelihood of the occurrence of subclinical disease.

Early detection of problems and routine screening for the presence of subclinical diseases or reduced organ function are important clinical objectives in the management of older animals. Performance of a full physical examination and blood and urine tests at regular intervals is useful because it helps to:

(1) detect problems early to increase the chance of successful intervention to delay or prevent the onset and/or progression of disease;
(2) provide base 'normals' for the individual against which future measurements can be compared;
(3) demonstrates a caring attitude towards the patient and helps to move the practice away from providing a fire brigade service (only providing treatment at times of illness) to one of providing a comprehensive preventative medicine programme.

Health screening of older patients is important particularly before the administration of a general anaesthetic, the use of a therapeutic agent with narrow margins of safety, or the administration of drugs that require normal hepatic, renal or cardiac function. Modification of drug dosage may be necessary in patients with impaired organ function with or without evidence of subclinical disease.

An annual vaccination programme provides the opportunity to perform a full physical examination and would be an ideal time to recommend further screening tests although for some animals, particularly those that have a medical history of serious illness, checks should probably be more frequent – say every 6 months. Unfortunately with many owners their compliance with an annual vaccination programme deteriorates with time.

Some practices prefer to offer a geriatric screening programme separate from the usual routine vaccination/worming and flea control consultations – and this may have merit in that it allows the programme to be offered as a 'special' service. My personal experience of running a geriatric clinic is that some owners will gladly pay for screening tests whereas others will not.

Some practices claim that the best results may be obtained by offering the initial consultation free of charge as a 'lost-leader' with the costs of providing the service being borne by the follow-up work (e.g. dental work, or the implementation of a dietary programme) that is often generated as a direct result of the screening programme.

As a student I was taught to perform laboratory and other investigative tests only when they were indicated from the history and physical examination. However, my personal experience since graduation has been that serious conditions may be missed by selectively omitting tests from a screening profile, and I now prefer to perform a complete screen whenever possible (see Table 10.1). Fortunately technological advances have resulted in a significant decrease in the cost of laboratory testing, and sometimes it is actually cheaper to perform a full profile screen than to request a few specific tests. In my opinion it is good practice to include a wide range of tests in a routine screening programme.

Radiography is an important aid to diagnosis in geriatric animals (see Chapter 9) but the potential health hazards and the need to administer a general anaesthetic to most animals preclude it from being included in a routine geriatric screening programme unless it is indicated by the presence of a clinical problem. In the future survey ultrasonography may be useful in a geriatric screening programme.

10.2 HISTORY

A full clinical history should be obtained from the previous medical records and the owner. It is important to ascertain whether the presenting signs are sudden in onset, a predictable sequel to a problem earlier in life or the manifestation of an insidious, chronic disease process.

Table 10.1 Geriatric screening programme.

	Comments
Full detailed history	
Full physical examination	Including a full neurological examination and ophthalmoscopy
Haematology	Haemoglobin, red cell count, PCV (HCT ratio), MCV, MCH, MCHC, white cell count, differential and platelets Screen report
Blood chemistry	Urea, creatinine, urea: creatinine ratio, ALT, AP, gamma-GT, bilirubin, total protein, albumin, globulin, bile acids, glucose, amylase, lipase, sodium, potassium, sodium:potassium ratio, chloride, calcium, phosphorus, calcium:phosphorus ratio, AST, CK, LDH, cholesterol, triglycerides
Urinalysis	Specific gravity, pH, glucose, protein, bilirubin, sediment (cells, crystals, casts) Water deprivation test – under observed conditions only
Blood pressure	Direct or indirect methods – non-invasive preferable, e.g. Dynamap
Hormone assay	Thyroid and parathyroid hormone. Basal cortisol (with low dose dexamethasone and/or ACTH stimulation tests if indicated) and possibly vitamin D estimation
Glomerular Filtration rate	Indirect measurement using labelled technetium
ECG/EMG/ERG	When indicated by the presence of cardiac or metabolic disorders (ECG): weakness or neuromuscular disease (EMG): vision problems (ERG)
Other tests	In the future the following screening tests might be useful: • urine lysozyme concentration • 2,3 DPG estimation • blood viscosity measurement • red cell deformity • survey ultrasonography

PCV, packed cell volume; HCT ratio, haematocrit ratio; MCV, mean corpuscular volume; MCH, mean corpuscular haemoglobin; MCHC, mean corpuscular haemoglobin concentration; ALT, alanine aminotransferase; AP, alkaline phosphatase; gamma-GT, δ glutamyl transferase; AST, aspartate aminotransferase; CK, creatine kinase; LDH, lactate dehydrogenase; ACTH, adrenocorticotrophic hormone; ECG, electrocardiogram; EMG, electromyogram; ERG, electroretinogram; DPG, 2,3-diphosphoglycerate.

Older animals frequently have a complex history and inexperienced clinicians often find it difficult to assess the significance of specific findings from the history in relation to current presenting signs. The temptation is to assume that clinical signs associated with a single organ system must be related, when in fact they usually are not. It is important that the previous medical record is examined in some detail in case there is a trend to suggest an on-going chronic disease process, and this is facilitated by the use of:

(1) a comprehensive recording system for clinical information
(2) standardisation of clinical record keeping by clinical members of staff
(3) the use of computers to store clinical records – because the records are less likely to be lost or damaged and are easy to retrieve in chronological order and in a standard format.

Owners may have difficulty in recalling the full history of geriatric patients, and often they are not as forthcoming about signs of illness which they consider to be 'normal' for an old animal. A decreasing response to visual stimuli is commonly reported and yet poor vision may be caused by a plethora of disease processes and is not necessarily just part of the ageing process.

10.3 PHYSICAL EXAMINATION

Many older animals will have concomitant disease and so it is important to perform a full clinical examination and not just focus on the problem(s) raised by the animal owner. In particular evidence should be sought for the presence of cardiac, respiratory, hepatic or renal dysfunction which are all common in advancing age, and for external evidence of internal disease. Dermatologists frequently refer to the skin as an indicator of general health and this can certainly be true in older animals (see Table 10.2).

Table 10.2 Skin signs in old animals as indicators of internal disease.

Sign	Possible age-related disease association
Alopecia – bilaterally symmetrical	Ovarian imbalance in mature bitches: • naturally occurring in entire bitches – may be associated with cystic or neoplastic ovaries *or* • in bitches spayed before first oestrus – sometimes also associated with urinary incontinence Sertoli cell tumour of the testis – more common in retained testicles Seminomas – rare Interstitial (Leydig) cell tumours – rare Testosterone-responsive alopecia – rare. Seen in middle-aged to old entire or castrated dogs
Alopecia, thinning of the skin, seborrhoea, pyoderma	Hepatocutaneous syndrome (due to cirrhosis) Diabetes mellitus

Table 10.2 Continued

Sign	Possible age-related disease association
Non-pruritic bilaterally symmetrical alopecia, cutaneous calcification, other skin changes, e.g. macules.	Hyperadrenocorticism (Cushing's syndrome)
Pyoderma	Hypothyroidism Hyperadrenocorticism Compromised immunecompetence
Vulval-fold pyoderma	Obesity Urinary incontinence
Callus formation over bony prominences	Commonly seen in older animals, particularly large breed dogs which lie on rough surfaces Hypothyroidism
Interdigital cysts (pyoderma)	Autoimmune disease Immune-deficiency Hypothyroidism
Generalised folliculitis, cellulitis, furunculosis	General debilitation Hypothyroidism Compromised immunecompetence
Dry, dull, brittle hair coat. Patchy alopecia; loss of coat pigment; hyperkeratosis and hyperpigmentation of skin	Protein deficiency: ● nutritional deficiency ● protein-losing disease
Dull, dry coat with scaling. Patchy alopecia and seborrhoea. Sometimes patches of acute moist dermatitis	Fat deficiency: ● nutritional deficiency ● exocrine pancreatic insufficiency ● liver disease ● small intestine disease
Cutaneous lesions with multisystem involvement, e.g. polyarthritis, glomerulonephritis, thrombocytopenia, polymyositis, fever, seizures	Systemic lupus erythematosus (SLE)
Paronychia	Diabetes mellitus, SLE or other autoimmune disorder
Xanthoma	Diabetes mellitus
Seborrhoea	Hypothyroidsim Hyperadrenocorticism Diabetes mellitus Sex-hormone related Nutritional deficiency Liver disease Renal disease Intestinal disease – malabsorption Exocrine pancreatic insufficiency Neoplasia
Lick granuloma	Behavioural disorder/psychogenic Arthrosis

Greying of the hair – particularly around the face and muzzle is common with advancing age. Neoplasia of the skin is also common in older animals (see Chapter 6).

A full neurological examination is necessary to identify signs of primary or secondary neurological deficit or increased neurological responsiveness. Both the peripheral and central nervous systems should be examined. See Chapter 3 and Wheeler (1989) for further details.

Ophthalmoscopic examination may reveal evidence of increased tortuosity of retinal blood vessels or even of subclinical retinal haemorrhages typical of hypertensive patients. Sudden onset blindness due to retinal detachment (often bilateral) is a more severe manifestation of hypertension and is seen in the presence of renal failure.

Blood and urinalysis should form part of a comprehensive screening programme because quite simple and inexpensive tests can provide invaluable information to assist the clinician. However there are many pitfalls in taking laboratory samples and in interpreting laboratory results and the reader is advised to consult an authoritative text on the subject such as that by Bush (1991).

10.4 HAEMATOLOGY

The purpose of conducting a haematological screen is to identify abnormal parameters such as packed cell volume (PCV) or haemoglobin concentration, increased or reduced red or white cell numbers, altered red or white blood cell morphology, or an abnormal platelet count that may indicate the presence of disorders such as:

(1) anaemia
(2) dehydration
(3) myeloproliferative disorders
(4) immunosuppression
(5) infection.

Packed cell volume (PCV, haematocrit index)

Cat   Normal range: 0.30–0.45 l/l (30–45%)

Dog   Normal range: 0.37–0.66 l/l (48–66%)

A low PCV indicates the presence of anaemia with consequential reduction in oxygen carrying capacity in the blood – which may be particularly harmful in older animals in which tissues may be particularly sensitive to local hypoxia.

A high PCV usually indicates the presence of dehydration. Many authors consider that older animals are in a state of relative dehydration – and this is certainly likely in the presence of polyuric syndromes such as diabetes, renal failure and hyperadrenocorticism.

Red blood cell count

Cat   Normal range: $5–10 \times 10^{12}/l$

Dog   Normal range: $5.5–9.5 \times 10^{12}/l$

Low red blood cell (erythrocyte) numbers usually indicates the presence of anaemia. High red cell counts usually indicate the presence of dehydration – and only occasionally true polycythaemia.

Haemoglobin

Cat   Normal range: 8–15 g/dl

Dog   Normal range: 12–23 g/dl

High haemoglobin concentrations usually indicate the presence of dehydration, and occasionally polycythaemia.

Low haemoglobin concentrations usually indicate the presence of anaemia.

Mean corpuscular volume (MCV)

Cat   Normal range: 39–55 fl

Dog   Normal range: 60–77 fl

High MCV values may be caused by abnormally large, immature erythrocytes and is seen in regenerative anaemia (see below), myeloproliferative disorders, and rarely in macrocytic anaemia.

About 50% of cats with hyperthyroidism may have a high MCV.

Low MCV values are seen when red cell size is small such as is caused by chronic haemorrhage and occasionally iron deficiency or feline haemobartonella.

Mean corpuscular haemoglobin concentration (MCHC)

Cat   Normal range: 30–36 g/dl

Dog   Normal range: 32–36 g/dl

Low MCHC values are seen with hypochromic cells (due to iron deficiency secondary to chronic inflammatory disease, chronic infection and neoplasia), and in regenerative anaemia. Protein-losing conditions may also lead to protein deficiency and low MCHC values.

Erythrocyte sedimentation rate (ESR)

Has to be corrected according to PCV measurement (see Bush 1991).

Cat   Normal range: 0–12 mm/h

Dog   Normal range: 0–5 mm/h

A high ESR is seen in acute generalised infections (e.g. endocarditis), inflammatory diseases (e.g. peritonitis, pericarditis and pleuritis), rheumatoid arthritis, chronic pyometra, malignant neoplasia, renal failure, hypoproteinaemia, hypothyroidism, hyperadrenocorticism.

A low ESR (negative after correction for PCV) is seen in haemolytic anaemia.

Many of the red cell abnormalities reported will indicate the presence of anaemia and it is important to attempt to interpret the results accurately (Table 10.3).

Table 10.3 Types of anaemia.

Cause	Acute/chronic	Classification
Haemorrhage	Acute or chronic	Regenerative
Haemolytic	Acute or chronic	Regenerative
Hypoproliferative	Chronic	Non-regenerative

Regenerative anaemia (responsive as evidenced by the production of reticulocytes which are released into the circulation) occurs after haemorrhage or haemolysis. Non-regenerative anaemia is commonly associated with thrombocytopenia and myeloproliferative diseases (Table 10.4).

Table 10.4 Causes of anaemia in geriatric patients.

Type of anaemia	Likely causes in old animals
Haemolytic anaemia	Immune mediated Disseminated intravascular coagulation (DIC) Hypophosphataemia Neoplasia – especially myeloproliferative and lymphoproliferative tumours and splenic haemangiosarcoma
Non-regenerative anaemia	Myeloproliferative disorders Chronic inflammatory disease: • Chronic pyometra Neoplasia FeLV Inadequate erythropoeitin: • Chronic renal failure • Chronic liver disease Endocrine disorders: • Hypothyroidism • Hypoadrenocorticism
Haemorrhagic anaemia	Trauma Thrombocytopenia Liver failure Neoplasia (especially haemangiosarcoma) Infection Gastrointestinal ulceration Urinary tract haemorrhage Poisoning

Platelet count

Cat   Normal range: $300–700 \times 10^9/l$

Dog   Normal range: $200–500 \times 10^9/l$

Animals with obvious clinical signs of haemorrhage or with a regenerative anaemia on routine screening should have their platelet count monitored. However it is a useful examination to include in a routine screen because of the number of chronic, subclinical conditions which can affect circulating platelets.

A reduced number of platelets (thrombocytopenia) occurs due to decreased production, increased destruction or loss from the body circulation and is seen in bone marrow disease, uraemia, toxaemia, infection, hypoadrenocorticism, DIC, immune-mediated disorders, myeloproliferative disorders, haemorrhage and splenomegaly.

An increased number of platelets (thrombocytosis) occurs due to excessive production rate or decreased removal from the circulation and is seen in postsplenectomy, in acute or chronic infections, inflammatory disease, drug induced, some myeloproliferative disorders (most cause thrombocytopenia) or malignant neoplasia.

Abnormal red cell morphology

Occasionally laboratories will report abnormally appearing red blood cells and the appearance can be associated with specific clinical problems (see Table 10.5)

Table 10.5 Abnormal red cells and their clinical associations.

Abnormality reported	Likely associations
Crenation	Uraemia
Burr cells (severe crenation)	Severe uraemia Disseminated intravascular coagulation (DIC)
Spur cells	Canine splenic haemangiosarcoma/ haemangioma Liver disease: • Hyperbilirubinaemia • Portosystemic shunts
Leptocytes (thin flat erythorcytes)	Renal failure Liver disease: obstructive Hypothyroidism
Schistocytes (erythrocyte fragments)	DIC Malignant neoplasia, e.g. haemangiosarcomas
Teardrop/oval erythrocytes	Myeloproliferative disorders
Rouleau formation	Hypoproteinaemia due inflammatory or neoplastic disease
Nucleated red blood cells	Regenerative anaemia Myeloproliferative disorders Liver disease
Macrocytes	Hyperthyroidism (feline)
Microcytes	Iron deficiency secondary to chronic blood loss
Heinz bodies	Intestinal disease (cats)
Howell–Jolly bodies	Splenic tumours (dogs)

White blood cell count

Cat   Normal range: $3.5–19.5 \times 10^9/l$

Dog   Normal range: $6–17 \times 10^9/l$

The total white blood cell count is a measure of all types of white cell. High counts (leukocytosis) are almost always due to an increased number of neutrophils (neutrophilia) which occurs in the presence of infection, lymphoproliferative disorders, tissue necrosis, inflammation, hyperthyroidism, and as a side-effect of endogenous or exogenous steroids.

A low total white cell count (leucopenia) is usually due to neutropenia and is seen in the presence of infection (especially in early septicaemia and most of the common canine and feline viral infections), bone marrow cancer and uraemia.

Differential white cell count

The differential count provides the clinician with additional information upon which to interpret the laboratory findings.

Neutrophils
Cat

Juvenile cells (band cells)   Normal range: $0–0.3 \times 10^9/l$ (0–3%)
Adult cells   Normal range: $2.5–12.5 \times 10^9/l$ (35–75%)

Dog

Juvenile cells (band cells)   Normal range: $0–0.3 \times 10^9/l$ (0–3%)
Adult cells   Normal range: $2–11.5 \times 10^9/l$ (60–70%)

In old animals high neutrophil counts (neutrophilia) are most often associated with inflammation, infection, the presence of exogenous or endogenous corticosteroids, stress and some forms of myeloproliferative disorder (e.g. lymphosarcoma).

Low neutrophil counts (neutropenia) are most often associated with bacterial, viral or protozoal infections, immune-mediated disorders, testicular neoplasia, uraemia and bone marrow disease.

Large numbers of juvenile band cells (a so-called 'shift to the left') is usually associated with the presence of infection (particularly septicaemia), inflammation or regenerative anaemia. It is also associated with toxoplasmosis and dirofilaria infections – both of which are rare in the UK.

Eosinophils
Cat   Normal range: $0–0.5 \times 10^9/l$ (2–12%)

Dog   Normal range: $0.1–1.25 \times 10^9/l$ (2–10%)

High eosinophil counts (eosinophilia) are associated with allergies, parasitism, systemic eosinophilic syndrome in cats, hypoadrenocorticism, and infection, e.g. pyometra in cats and dogs.

Low eosinophil counts (eosinopenia) are associated with stress, hyperadrenocorticism and acute infection or inflammation. Eosinopenia has also been reported to occur in old dogs as part of the ageing process.

Basophils

Cat   Normal range: Rare

Dog   Normal range: Rare

Basophils are rarely seen on blood smears from cats and dogs. When present they are usually associated with allergic reactions. They are also seen associated with hyperlipoproteinaemia in dogs due to diabetes, liver disease, hyperadrenocorticism and nephrosis.

Monocytes

Cat   Normal range: $0.1–0.85 \times 10^9/l$ (1–4%)

Dog   Normal range: $0.15–1.35 \times 10^9/l$ (3–10%)

Only small numbers are usually seen in cat and dog blood. High monocyte counts are associated with hyperadrenocorticism, exogenous or endogenous steroids, and stress, inflammation, infection, immune-mediated tissue damage and malignancy. In fact any condition in which tissue damage is a feature.

Monocytosis is also reported to occur in old dogs as part of the ageing process.

Lymphocytes

Cat   Normal range: $1.5–7 \times 10^9/l$ (20–55%)

Dog   Normal range: $0.8–4.8 \times 10^9/l$ (12–30%)

In old animals high lymphocyte (lymphocytosis) counts are most likely associated with lymphocytic leukaemia or lymphosarcoma, stress, FIV infection, chronic immunestimulation or hypoadrenocorticism.

Hyperthyroid cats treated with methimazole or carbimazole may also develop lymphocytosis.

Low lymphocyte counts (lymphopenia) are usually associated with the effects of steroids (exogenous or endogenous), acute systemic infections, neoplasia of the lymphatic system, other lymphatic disease (including loss of lymph) and chronic renal failure. Atrophy of lymphatics is reported to occur in old age leading to lymphopenia.

Abnormal white cell morphology

Abnormal white cells are sometimes seen on blood smears:

(1) Mast cells may occur in the circulation following trauma or acute inflammation, and also in the presence of mast cell tumours.

(2) Lymphoblasts are seen in lymphoproliferative diseases, e.g. leukaemia.
(3) Macrophages are seen in the presence of bacterial infection.
(4) Juvenile white blood cells are seen in association with myeloproliferative diseases.
(5) Inclusion bodies may occur in lymphocytes, neutrophils or red blood cells following canine distemper virus infection. Various protozoa, fungi, and bacteria can be seen as intracellular infections – though most are rare in the UK.

10.5 BLOOD CHEMISTRY

Blood chemistry tests are an important part of a screening programme in older animals because they are particularly helpful in the detection of subclinical organ damage or functional failure.

Blood urea nitrogen (BUN)

Elevation of blood urea nitrogen (BUN) concentrations may be caused by many different things including pre-renal and post-renal factors and should not be considered diagnostic of primary renal disease in all cases. Additional blood biochemistry and urinalysis are necessary to evaluate fully the cause of high BUN concentrations. To eliminate dietary factors BUN should be performed on blood collected after 12 hours starvation.

Cat   Normal Range: 5–11 mmol/l

Dog   Normal range: 2.5–7 mmol/l

In old animals undergoing routine screening a high BUN may indicate the presence of:

Pre-renal causes

- dehydration
- increased catabolism
- hyperthyroidism
- intestinal haemorrhage
- necrosis
- hypoadrenocorticism
- hypoalbuminaemia.

Renal

- chronic renal failure or other renal disease
- nephrocalcinosis
- neoplasia.

Post-renal

- calculi
- neoplasia
- prostatic disease.

Cats are obligate carnivores and have liver enzyme systems for protein metabolism which do not down-regulate in the presence of reduced protein intake in the diet. As a consequence of this, and of the large number of clinical conditions that can lead to catabolism, a high BUN, muscle wastage and weight loss are common features in old cats. In fact, almost any major organ system disorder is accompanied by severe catabolism and loss of lean body mass in the cat.

Low BUN concentrations are seen in animals on low protein rations or in the presence of liver failure or acquired portosystemic shunts.

Plasma creatinine

Cat   Normal range: 40–130 µmol/l

Dog   Normal range: 40–130 µmol/l

Unlike BUN, plasma creatinine concentrations are unaffected by other systemic factors and because it is exclusively excreted via the kidneys high concentrations indicate reduced renal function whatever the primary cause. Creatinine is therefore a more useful test for renal function than BUN.

Urea: creatinine ratio

The normal ratio of plasma urea to creatinine is 0.08 or less. Some authors have suggested that this ratio can be used to predict the rate of progression of renal failure.

Serum alanine aminotransferase (ALT)

Hepatocyte damage releases the enzyme ALT and high concentrations are therefore indicative of active liver cell damage – whatever the primary cause. It is not a test that measures liver function, as only a small area of liver may be damaged to get significant increases in ALT – usually within 4–5 days. Even very high ALT concentrations can be followed by complete recovery by the liver.

Myocarditis can also result in an increase in ALT, but this is uncommon.

Alkaline phosphatase (ALP)

Alkaline phosphatase isoenzymes have been identified from various organs including the liver, bone, gastrointestinal tract, and kidney, and there is a specific isoenzyme produced in response to steroids in dogs. Increased ALP concentrations are usually associated with liver (particularly bile outflow obstruction) or bone disease (particularly tumours with new bone production as well as destruction or renal hyperparathyroidism).

ALP concentrations are increased in 90% of feline hyperthyroid cases.

Aspartate aminotransferase (AST)

Occurs in skeletal and cardiac muscle and in liver.

It is most helpful in identifying muscle damage (with creatine kinase) particularly myositis, and occasionally for cardiomyopathies.

Creatine kinase (CK)

Creatine kinase isoenzymes occur in skeletal and cardiac muscle and in the brain. It is most useful as an indicator of muscle damage.

It has been reported that old animals have lower concentrations.

10.6 URINALYSIS

Specific gravity

The single most important screening test for renal insufficiency is urine specific gravity, which can be measured using an hydrometer or refractometer. The latter are in common use and give reliable results.

Cat   Normal range: 1.035–1.060

Dog   Normal range: 1.015–1.045

A pale coloured urine with a low specific gravity indicates increased water excretion (polyuria) and is seen in many of the clinical conditions which are common in older cats and dogs, e.g. renal failure, diabetes, hyperadrenocorticism (dogs), canine pyometra, hypercalcaemia, and liver disease.

A high urine specific gravity indicates urine concentration and may be caused by decreased renal perfusion as in shock, dehydration or cardiac disease.

pH

The acidity or alkalinity of urine is usually measured in dog and cat urine by using test strips but more accurate results can be obtained by using a pH meter. The normal range for the dog and cat is 5.5–7. Urine pH is diet sensitive, with high protein rations causing an acidic urine. In the post-prandial period following a meal there is an alkaline tide during which the pH becomes less acidic. Table 10.6 lists the causes of abnormal urine pH.

Table 10.6 Causes of abnormal urine pH.

Urine pH	Causes
Acidic (less than pH 5.5)	Respiratory acidosis
	Shock
	Vomiting or diarrhoea
	Ketoacidosis
	Azotaemia
	Protein catabolism
	Drugs/diets causing acidosis
Alkaline (pH greater than 7)	Respiratory alkalosis
	Vomiting
	Urinary tract infection
	Postprandial alkaline tide
	Plant-based rations

Urine protein

Most proteins are usually retained in the circulation and are not filtered through the glomerulus into the urine, however in dog urine concentrations of protein of 0.5 g/l are normal. Most of this protein (which is mainly albumin) originates from the kidney itself and the lower urinary tract and has not been filtered through the glomeruli. Care is needed in interpreting protein concentrations in urine because this can be affected by the dilution effects of polyuria.

Test strips are commonly used in veterinary practice and these are more sensitive to albumin than to other proteins. A more useful measure is 24-hour urinary protein loss but this requires collection of all voided urine over a 24 hour period which is not practical without access to a metabolism cage. Normal urine protein loss can be up to 30 mg/kg body weight per day.

Excessive concentrations of protein in urine (above 10 g/l) are the result of renal disease (various types – but mainly chronic renal failure or glomerular disease), inflammatory disease, hyperproteinaemia (renal threshold is 100 g/l plasma protein), haemorrhage, haemaglobinaemia or myoglobinaemia.

Glucose

Glucosuria is usually associated with diabetes mellitus, but is also seen in hyperadrenocorticism, hyperthyroidism, chronic liver disease, renal failure, feline lower urinary tract disease and phaechromocytoma.

Crystalluria

Examination of urine sediment (in a fresh sample) can be very useful to detect abnormal cells (e.g. blood cells, cancer cells) and crystals. If possible the urine should be fresh as crystals precipitate out as urine cools and other changes occur with changes in acidity or alkalinity.

Struvite, oxalate, urate and cystine crystals may be associated with urolithiasis and sometimes with primary or secondary urinary tract infection. Ammonium urate crystalluria occurs with liver disease and portocaval shunts. Calcium containing crystals may increase in the presence of hyperparathyroidism.

REFERENCES AND FURTHER READING

Bush, B.M. (1991) *Interpretation of Laboratory Results for Small Animal Clinicians.* Blackwell Scientific Publications, Oxford.
Wheeler, S.J. (1989) *Manual of Small Animal Neurology.* British Small Animal Veterinary Association, Cheltenham.

INDEX